Cancer Navigation

Cancer Navigation

*Charting the Path Forward for Low-Income
Women of Color*

ANJANETTE A. WELLS
VETTA L. SANDERS THOMPSON
WILL ROSS
CAROL CAMP YEAKEY
SHERI R. NOTARO

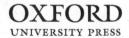

OXFORD
UNIVERSITY PRESS

Oxford University Press is a department of the University of Oxford. It furthers the University's objective of excellence in research, scholarship, and education by publishing worldwide. Oxford is a registered trade mark of Oxford University Press in the UK and certain other countries.

Published in the United States of America by Oxford University Press
198 Madison Avenue, New York, NY 10016, United States of America.

Library of Congress Cataloging-in-Publication Data
Names: Anjanette A. Wells, author.
Title: Cancer navigation : charting the path forward for low income women of color /
Anjanette A. Wells, Vetta L. Sanders Thompson, Will Ross, Carol Camp Yeakey, Sheri R. Notaro.
Description: New York, NY : Oxford University Press, [2022] | Includes
bibliographical references and index.
Identifiers: LCCN 2021034564 (print) | LCCN 2021034565 (ebook) |
ISBN 9780190672867 (paperback) | ISBN 9780190672881 (epub) |
ISBN 9780197626191
Subjects: LCSH: Cancer in women—Social aspects. | Cancer in
women—Prevention. | Cancer in women—Economic aspects. | Poor
women—Medical care—United States. | Health literacy.
Classification: LCC RC281.W65 A55 2022 (print) | LCC RC281.W65 (ebook) |
DDC 362.19699/40082—dc23
LC record available at https://lccn.loc.gov/2021034564
LC ebook record available at https://lccn.loc.gov/2021034565

DOI: 10.1093/OSO/9780190672867.001.0001

1 3 5 7 9 8 6 4 2

Printed by Marquis, Canada

This volume is dedicated to those marginalized women of color, at risk for and suffering from the ravages of cancer, and to those who provide support and comfort for them.

Contents

Acknowledgments   ix

INTRODUCTION   1
Purpose and Summary of This Book   1
    Module I.1: Cancer 101   6
        Cancer Among Low-Income Women of Color   7
        What Is Cancer?   7
        What's Known and Unknown About Cancer Among Women of Color?   8
        Types of Cancer   9
        Causes of Cancer and Risk Factors   9
        Screening Recommendations   11
Module I.2: Chronic Care Conceptual Model   19
Conclusion   27

1. Interpersonal, Community, and Population Communication and
   Engagement   30
    Module 1.1: Cancer Communication   30
        Health Literacy: Literacy in Support of Health   31
        Health Communication for Colorectal Cancer Screening and Treatment
           of Low-Income and Racial and Ethnic Communities   33
        Conclusion   39
    Module 1.2: Recognizing and Assessing Adherence Barriers and Stressors   43
        Adherence Barriers and Facilitators: Breast Cancer Treatment Among
           African American Women   45
        Adherence Barriers and Stressors   47
        Case 1: Ms. Smith   50
        Case 2: Maria   52
        Poverty Profiles of Low-Income Women   54
    Module 1.3: Culturally Competent Communication, Assessment,
    and Engagement   71
        What Is Cultural Competency?   72
        Why Is Cultural Competency Important to the Practice with Low-Income
           Women of Color?   72
        Cultural Competency in Practice   73
        Applying Cultural Competence to Intersectional Identities and Needs   74
        Concepts of Difference in Health   75
        Social Determinants of Health   77
        National Standards for Culturally and Linguistically Appropriate Services   77
        Other Important Cultural Competency Concepts   77

2. Intervention and Strategies Across the Cancer Continuum   85
    Module 2.1: Patient Navigation   85
        What Is Patient Navigation?   86
        Training for Patient Navigators   87

Starting the Patient Navigation Process   88
Problem Solving   89
Information   91
Motivation   92
Behavioral Skills   97
Adapting Patient Navigation   97
Conclusion   100
Module 2.2: Survivorship Care Plans   112
Cancer Survivors   112
Cancer Survivorship Care Plans   113
Adapted SCP   117
Module 2.3: Clinical Trial Uptake: Additional Options for Treatment   123
Underrepresentation by Specific Subgroups   123
Barriers to Clinical Trial Participation   125
Storyboard Illustrations   127

3. Evaluation of Cancer Interventions and Programs   136
Module 3.1: Outcomes and Assessing Intervention Efforts   136
CDC Model for Program Evaluation   139
Concluding the Evaluation   147
Summary   148
Module 3.2: Community-Based Participatory Research   149
What Is CBPR?   149
What Is Community?   150
Who Is a Community Stakeholder?   151
Social Ecological Model   152
Phases in Conducting CBPR   152
Summary   163

CONCLUSION   167
Summary of the Introduction   167
Summary of Chapter 1   168
Summary of Chapter 2   169
Summary of Chapter 3   170
Future Research   170
Conclusion   171

Index   175

Acknowledgments

No volume is written alone. First, the co-authors wish to acknowledge the first author, Professor Anjanette A. Wells, whose original work on cancer prevention provided the intellectual impetus for this project. Second, a special thank you to coauthors Vetta Sanders Thompson, Will Ross, Carol Camp Yeakey, and Sheri Notaro, who worked collaboratively and seamlessly to break down academic disciplinary boundaries and foster cross-disciplinary and interprofessional dialog. This book is a tangible result of these collaborations. Thank you to Andy Meade (from Meaden Creative), Richard May, III, Nicole Volpenhein, and Nadia Alam for your creativity in designing the graphics and illustrations with so much sensitivity and rich complexity; we sincerely appreciate your beautiful and thoughtful designs. Similarly, we thank our students, in particular Angela Bird, Nadia Alam, Jossie Jones, and Lauren Styczynski, for their assistance assembling data, editing, and compiling references. Special thanks to Hanlin Zhou for the careful attention in researching and generating the GIS mapping. We also need to acknowledge the Oxford University Press editorial staff, including Dana Bliss and his team; thank you for your continued patience, confidence, comprehensive vision, and guidance through all aspects of this publication process. Further, we owe a tremendous debt of gratitude to the marginalized women of color in our study who allowed us into their lives at a most vulnerable and challenging time. We applaud you for your courage and strength. It is to you that this volume is dedicated. Last but not least, we wish to thank our close friends and infinitely patient families who have endured our need to spend time away from gatherings on revising drafts and setting up conference calls in an attempt to capture the right words to further serious discussion on such timely and sensitive subject matter. Of course, the final product is our own creation and we accept full responsibility for its contents. To all healthcare providers, we trust that we have provided tools and strategies that can be useful in your passionate and compassionate work to improve health equity for low-income women of color.

While we have attempted to provide and illuminate pathways forward for low-income women as they navigate the travails of cancer, we can only hope that our work is of some small comfort to them and to those who care for them. Any omissions or shortcomings in this volume are ours alone. We hope that this volume becomes an invaluable resource for patient navigators as they provide guidance and support for marginalized populations of cancer patients. We trust that we have rendered the ensuring pages with the sensitivity, sincerity, and honesty that low-income women of color, afflicted with cancer, deserve.

Introduction

Of all the forms of inequality, injustice in health is the most shocking and inhumane.

Dr. Martin Luther King, Jr. (1966)

Purpose and Summary of This Book

Being poor is a health risk (Wells et al., 2019). When we wrote *Poverty and Place: Cancer Prevention Among Low-Income Women of Color* in 2019, we demonstrated the potent forces of poverty and place and the prevalence of cancer among low-income women of color. That initial volume was the inspiration for this volume, entitled *Cancer Navigation: Charting the Path Forward for Low-Income Women of Color*. In *Poverty and Place*, we had academics and researchers in mind. Our purpose was to examine how and why racial and class disparities have become potent forces in health and longevity rates in the United States. Conducting original research drawn from North St. Louis, Missouri, and the river city of East St. Louis, Illinois, we sought to understand the combination of factors that facilitate or pose barriers to cancer treatment and adherence for marginalized low-income women of color.

We know that poverty is associated with a huge array of human ills, not the least of which is seriously undermining the health of impoverished people. Due to limited financial resources, the poor are recurrently subjected to environmental risks due to unavailability of suitable housing, are less well nourished, and have less knowledge about and are less able to access healthcare and appropriate health insurance. As a result, they consistently have a higher incidence of numerous illnesses and diseases. The diseases in turn can diminish already beleaguered household savings, reduce their ability to work, and further diminish their quality of life, thereby perpetuating or even increasing poverty. It has been established that the poor tend to suffer worse health and die at a younger age than their wealthier counterparts.

As documented in the American Cancer Society's annual "Cancer Facts and Figures" (2016), poverty remains one of the most potent carcinogens. A carcinogen is defined as any substance or agent that produces cancer or that causes cells to become cancerous by altering their genetic structure so that they multiply and become malignant. While non-Hispanic White females have a higher incidence of breast cancer, non-Hispanic African American women have a higher mortality rate (American Cancer Society, 2016). Similar reports by the American Cancer Society (2016) conclude that poverty is the initial contributing factor to cancer disparities among social groups and that racial differences in biological or inherited characteristics are less significant. The fact is that people living in poverty lack access to healthcare and endure greater pain, illness, and subsequent death (Heidary et al., 2013). One population that suffers acutely are low-income women of color, the focus of this volume.

Cancer Navigation. Anjanette A. Wells, Vetta L. Sanders Thompson, Will Ross, Carol Camp Yeakey, and Sheri R. Notaro, Oxford University Press. © Oxford University Press 2022. DOI: 10.1093/med/9780190672867.003.0001

While health disparities are based on real data, our broader focus is on those factors that increase health equity. As Rick Kittles noted:

> Health equity . . . focuses on . . . the incidence, prevalence, mortality and outcomes of diseases across various populations. You can stratify those populations in many ways: race, education, geography, socioeconomic status. Health equity explores ways in which we can engage and intervene to eliminate some of those differences that we see across populations. For example, black women are much more susceptible to triple-negative breast cancer . . . It's very clear that across any cancers there are various inequities in incidence and outcomes, and we're looking at ways that we can level that playing field. (Bonar, 2018)

It is the express intent of this volume to provide a strategic framework needed to impact and increase the health equity of all marginalized populations in general, but low-income women of color in particular.

Cancer Navigation: Charting the Path Forward for Low-Income Women of Color is intended to be a practical guide mainly for individuals who care about the health of low-income women of color and provide support and comfort to them. This book is to be used as a guidebook, an easily accessible, affordable, and quick reference resource. It may be useful for the busy U.S. healthcare providers who are passionately and compassionately working with marginalized women throughout the cancer continuum, from community preventive outreach to survivorship. Despite all of the evidence and research that went into *Poverty and Place*, our goal is to make sure that frontline helpers have a valuable resource at their disposal. This guide is meant for practitioners who spend time not only attempting to help women navigate their health and work through the often alienating healthcare system, but also assisting them in working through the hassles of daily life. Although there are limits on what providers can do, there is also great potential for doing more and doing it better. We often think we don't have time to provide compassion, yet we don't have time *not* to provide humane care. Passion and compassion in cancer care for low-income women of color is not an issue of pity or based solely on medical or scientific care; it is more an issue of social justice.

Capturing the social determinants of health is one way to advance social justice, for the issues are not just about the lack of financial resources but also involve structural racial barriers and implicit bias. What are the social determinants of health? They include unequal exposure to health-damaging conditions, influenced by social, economic, and political factors that impact individual and group differences in health status (Braveman & Gottlieb, 2014) rather than individual risk factors (such as behavioral risk factors or genetics). The World Health Organization suggests, "This unequal distribution of health-damaging experiences is not in any sense a 'natural' phenomenon but is the result of a toxic combination of poor social policies, unfair economic arrangements (where the already well-off and healthy become even richer and the poor who are already more likely to be ill become even poorer), and bad politics" (Commission on Social Determinants of Health, 2008, p. 1).

The COVID-19 pandemic reminds us of the extreme vulnerability of communities of color as well as the pathology of racism that makes the pathology of the coronavirus worse. Black America, indeed all communities of color in America, have become ground zero for COVID-19 (Chen & Krieger, 2020). Institutionalized racism has produced a system that drives disparities in health outcomes across lifetimes and generations. Higher levels of discrimination and bias are associated with elevated risk of a broad range of diseases, from higher levels of stress hormones, to high blood pressure, to obesity and early death. All of those underlying conditions put people of color in general, and low-income people of color in particular, at higher risk for bad outcomes from COVID-19. The nexus of higher unemployment rates, mass incarceration, chronic pre-existing medical issues, poor housing, homelessness, and less reliable access to quality healthcare exemplify the vulnerability of African Americans, indeed all persons of color, to increased viral transmission, infection, and death during a pandemic. Even worse, low-income persons of color are less likely to have the type of employment that will continue to pay if they don't physically come to work. Indeed, the ability to work from home, to practice social distancing, and to wear a mask without fear of being arrested or shot are forms of privilege that few persons of color enjoy (Blow, 2020).

The challenge for us in writing and compiling this book was to find a way for transdisciplinary providers to use it in the hustle-bustle of clinical practice. We have been cautious not to dilute the research or oversimplify complex issues into practical elements. This volume is meant to provide useful and practical strategies, many of them grounded in our research and experience. We wanted to convey just enough of the essential strategies to make the volume accessible, learnable, useful, and effective in a variety of healthcare and community settings with low-income women of color. We offer strategies that go beyond working with women in the abstract to considering the social determinants of health and contextual strategies that situate women in their environment and in the healthcare system, which can enhance the assistance and care that they receive. We are realistic. When you finish reading this book, you will not be an expert in some of the skills, nor will all of the tools and strategies be specifically customized to the women with whom you work. Rather, *Cancer Navigation: Charting the Path Forward for Low-Income Women of Color* is meant as an introduction and overview to familiarize you with this population and obtain a glimpse into their experiences and needs. We encourage you to do so with a nonjudgmental and open attitude.

As academics and researchers, we often spend hours working on scholarship that never gets translated into work with real clients or the very persons who need tangible and intangible resources. This book is our attempt to fill that gap. While this volume is focused on cancer and cancer navigation strategies that support treatment and recovery among low-income women of color, cancer can be used as an example for other illness domains requiring long-term care and support. In effect, this volume can be used as a model and framework for other illness domains.

In this setting, the list of providers, of those who deliver, supply, diagnose, and furnish assistance and care, is infinite: oncologists, primary care physicians, social workers, case managers, nurses, schedulers, medical assistants, patient navigators, community health workers, health advocates, community stakeholders, peer health coaches, health ambassadors, professors and teachers, intervention researchers, public health educators, students, husbands, partners, sisters, mothers, daughters, friends, grassroots community activists, cancer survivors, coworkers. These individuals do their very best to support, encourage, treat and motivate those living with cancer, but many do not have the resources, time, or support to access reference materials or receive training or preparation on how to work with cancer patients in a relatable and nonjudgmental way. This is why this volume, entitled *Cancer Navigation: Charting the Path Forward for Low-Income Women of Color*, was born.

In this volume, chapters are organized as modules to permit access to intervention and navigation information in a format that can be accessed in order, over time, or as discrete lessons accessed on an as-needed basis. We begin with a brief overview of cancer and a theory to guide navigators, lay health workers, or other support personnel new to cancer prevention, treatment, and survivorship support. Module I.1, entitled "Cancer 101," explains cancer as a collection of related diseases and provides some of the "known" and "unknown" facts about cancer among women of color. This chapter focuses upon the fact that lung, breast, colorectal, and cervical cancers are common among low-income women of color. The authors point out that while biological factors may account for some differences, social factors have a greater influence on disparities for a number of reasons (National Cancer Institute, 2018). An explanation of risk factors, behaviors to reduce risk, and screening and early detection methods is provided. The chapter ends with a glossary of cancer-related terms that will be useful to cancer patients and cancer navigators as well.

The chronic care model (CCM) provides the overarching theoretical framework for *Cancer Navigation: Charting the Path Forward for Low-Income Women of Color*. It is introduced in Module I.2. The CCM is a multifaceted, evidence-based framework for enhancing care delivery by identifying essential components of the healthcare system that can be modified to support high-quality, patient-centered chronic disease management. The CCM provides a systematic approach to practice transformation. Used in a variety of healthcare settings to guide systematic and individual improvement in chronic illness care, the CCM operates with a strategy of bringing together the patient, the provider, and system interventions necessary to accomplish the overall goal of improving care for chronic illness. The model consists of six interrelated and intersecting components of healthcare delivery:

1. Health system support, including culture, organizations, and mechanisms to promote safe, high-quality care
2. Clinical information systems to organize patient and population data
3. Delivery system design for clinical care and self-management support, including team care
4. Decision support based on evidence and patients' preferences and needs
5. Patient self-management support to enable patients to manage their health and health care
6. Community resources to mobilize patient resources.

Why is the CCM important in our effort to present key cancer navigation strategies for low-income women of color? Chronic diseases and their management are quickly becoming one of the largest elements of primary care. The CCM has been used widely for many years in a variety of settings, though many providers have struggled to implement the model in a way that is cost effective in both chronic care management and in practice improvement (Davy et al., 2015).

Chapter 1, "Interpersonal, Community and Population Communication and Engagement," provides an overview and examples of how various communication strategies and interventions can be used to support and improve screening and treatment adherence among low-income women. Standards for community-engaged strategies to facilitate development of plain-language communication and education materials that use visual composition, layout, and design to address and support health literacy are discussed. Health literacy tips for navigators and lay and community health workers are provided. Strategies to assess barriers and stressors that affect cancer prevention behaviors and treatment adherence frequently encountered by low-income women are described. Finally, the importance of including the patient's unique values, beliefs, and cultural practices in health education and behavior is discussed, with recommendations for application in cancer education and communication.

Chapter 2, "Intervention and Strategies Across the Cancer Continuum," includes individual (e.g., CBT-based interventions) and interpersonal (e.g., patient navigation) strategies, highlighting two well-known interventions: patient navigation and motivational interviewing (MI; Miller & Rollnick, 1991). In this chapter we use an approach that extends beyond "barrier/stressor reduction" techniques to include motivational skills to promote adherence. MI, a clinical intervention shown to improve motivation and increase medical adherence, can be used by patient navigators and other healthcare providers to improve timely cancer care and screening. MI is a collaborative and empowering approach effective at changing patients' health behaviors and improving their adherence to illness and disease management, through the use of patient-centered skills and strategies. This chapter presents an adapted MI, tailored to providers working with this population in busy healthcare practice settings and with patients who experience multiple adherence barriers and stressors. A graphic in this chapter summarizes the types of statements we often hear from women who are ambivalent about seeking care and matches these statements with examples of provider responses that can be used to evoke "change talk."

Survivorship care plans and additional options for treatment are also significant points of discussion in this chapter. Included as well are specific questions relevant to this population from mandated survivorship care plans, as a way to illustrate examples used in real-world practice. This chapter provides a graphic depicting the cancer trajectory model based on research from African American breast cancer survivors. The survivors discussed their experiences and offered advice for targeting needs at each cancer stage from screening to diagnosis, treatment, and then survivorship. The model illustrates the cyclical cancer course, with each quadrant representing a different phase in the cancer trajectory. The cancer trajectory model is different from other linear diagrams because it illustrates that the trajectory is not complete at the survivorship phase, but rather shows ongoing influences. Module 2.3 discusses the role of clinical trials in cancer treatment and factors that may affect participation of low-income women and racial and ethnic minorities. Communication and decision-making about clinical trial participation is discussed.

Chapter 4, "Evaluation of Cancer Interventions and Programs," discusses evidence-based public health practice in the evaluation of cancer interventions and programs. Most importantly, this chapter explores the evaluation of interventions within a health equity framework. Important to this discussion is intentionality—that is, taking into consideration whether the outcomes of programs and interventions differ for underrepresented or marginalized communities. Discussions of outcomes and the assessment of intervention efforts as well as community-based participatory research add to this important section on evaluation of cancer interventions and programs.

The book ends with a concluding section that summarizes the previous chapters and adds suggestions for future research.

We wish to thank all of the participants, community organizations, and institutions advocating for, treating, and supporting women living with cancer who have assisted us in our research. In addition, we are grateful for the tolerance, patience, and support of our families and loved ones as we have completed the previous and current volume.

We hope this volume becomes an invaluable resource for patient navigators as they provide guidance and support for marginalized populations of cancer patients. While we have attempted to provide and illuminate pathways forward for low-income women as they navigate the travails of cancer, we can only hope that our work is of some small comfort to them and to those who care for them. Any omissions or shortcomings in this volume are ours alone. We trust that we have rendered the ensuing pages with the sensitivity, sincerity, and honesty that low-income women of color, living with cancer, deserve.

References

American Cancer Society. (2016). Cancer facts and figures, US 2011–2016. https://www.cancer.org/content/dam/cancer-org/research/cancer-facts-and-statistics/annual-cancer-facts-and-figures/2016/cancer-facts-and-figures-2016.pdf

Bonar, S. (2018). Rick Kittles, Ph.D.: On a mission to eliminate health inequities. City of Hope. https://www.cityofhope.org/breakthroughs/rick-kittles-is-on-a-mission-to-eliminate-health-inequities

Braveman, P., & Gottlieb, L. (2014). The social determinants of health: It's time to consider the causes of the causes. *Public Health Reports, 129*(1_suppl2), 19–31.

Blow, C. (March 5, 2020). Covid-19's race and class warfare. *New York Times.*

Chen, J. T., & Krieger, N. (April 1, 2020). Revealing the unequal burden of COVID-19 by income, race/ethnicity, and household crowding: US county vs. ZIP code analyses. Harvard Center for Population and Development Studies. Working Paper, Volume 19, Number 1.

Commission on Social Determinants of Health (2008). Closing the gap in a generation: health equity through action on the social determinants of health. Final Report of the Commission on Social Determinants of Health. Geneva, World Health Organization. https://www.who.int/social_determinants/final_report/csdh_finalreport_2008.pdf

Davy, C., Bleasel, J., Liu, H., Tchan, M., Ponniah, S., & Brown, A. (2015). Effectiveness of chronic care models: Opportunities for improving healthcare practice and health outcomes: A systematic review. *BMC Health Services Research, 15*, 194. doi:10.1186/s12913-015-0854-8

Heidary, F., Rahimi, A., & Gharebaghi, R. (2013). Poverty as a risk factor in human cancers. *Iranian Journal of Public Health, 42*(3), 341–343.

Miller, W. R., & Rollnick, S. (1991) *Motivational interviewing: Preparing people to change addictive behavior.* Guilford Press.

National Cancer Institute. (2018). Cancer health disparities research. https://www.cancer.gov/research/areas/disparities

Wells, A., Thompson, V. L. S., Ross, W., Yeakey, C. C., & Notaro, S. R. (2019). *Poverty and place: Cancer prevention among low-income women of color.* Lexington Books.

Module I.1: Cancer 101

This module explains cancer as a collection of related diseases and provides some of the "known" and "unknown" facts about cancer among women of color. We focus on the fact that lung, breast, colorectal, and cervical cancers are common among low-income women of color. While the biological factors may account for some differences, social factors have a greater influence on disparities for a number of reasons (NIH, 2018). We

Table I.1 Cancer Knowledge Pretest

1.	T	F	NS	The most common types of cancer among low-income women of color are breast, cervical, colorectal, lung.
2.	T	F	NS	Breast cancer is the leading cancer in women.
3.	T	F	NS	Detecting cervical cancer begins with the Pap screening.
4.	T	F	NS	There is nothing that can be done to prevent cancer.
5.	T	F	NS	Smoking is the leading cause of lung cancer.

Circle your choice: true (T), false (F), or not sure (NS).

provide an explanation of risk factors, behaviors to reduce risk, and screening and early detection methods, as well as a glossary of cancer-related terms, which will be useful to cancer patients and healthcare providers alike.

Cancer Among Low-Income Women of Color

We begin our discussion of cancer among low-income women of color with a pretest for patient navigators and providers. This pretest (Table I.1) is used to measure your existing knowledge and understanding of the prevalence of cancer and cancer prevention. You can also develop and use a similar short pretest and posttest with your patients to provide immediate feedback about their understanding and increase awareness and knowledge, particularly when there are time restrictions on patient visits and increased patient workloads. The posttest (Table I.5) at the end of this module is used to evaluate knowledge gained from the content in this module, based on the four types of cancer that are most common among low-income women of color and their associated recommended screenings.

Before you can understand a problem and subsequently address it, you need to be able to define important terms and concepts related to that problem. For that reason, we thought it was critical to introduce several important terms that need to be understood. Table I.2 defines important terms related to cancer among low-income women of color.

What Is Cancer?

The term "cancer" refers to a collection of related diseases. All of these different types of cancer are similar in that they occur when some of the body's cells begin to divide without stopping and then spread to surrounding tissues. The human body is made up of cells, with different body parts having their own types of cells. When things are functioning properly, human cells grow and divide to provide the body with new cells as needed. Old and damaged cells die, and new cells replace them.

However, when cancer develops, the cycle of cell growth, death, and replacement is disrupted. Old cells survive instead of dying, and new cells form when they are not needed. Growths known as "tumors" form when extra cells divide without stopping. Many cancers form solid tumors, or masses of tissue; however, cancers of the blood do not form solid tumors (NIH, 2018).

Table I.2 Glossary of Cancer-Related Terms

Cancer disparities	"Differences in cancer outcomes among different population groups, which may include, but are not limited to, those characterized by race/ethnicity, ancestry, cultural factors, socioeconomic status, age, sexual orientation, geography, disability or other characteristics associated with social inequality or discrimination" (komen.org)
Barriers	Stressors, obstacles that prevent cancer screening or treatment adherence.
Federally Qualified Health Center	"A health center which qualifies for funding under Section 330 of the Public Health Service Act (PHS); qualifies for enhanced reimbursement from Medicare and Medicaid, as well as other benefits; serves an underserved population or area; offers a sliding scale fee; provides comprehensive services (on-site or by arrangement with another provider); has an ongoing quality assurance program; and has a governing board of directors" (www.fqhc.org/what-is-an-fqhc)
Oncologist	A medical practitioner qualified to diagnose and treat cancerous tumors
Social determinants	Economic and social conditions that influence individual and group differences in health status
Underserved	Disadvantaged populations such as low-income communities, under- or uninsured persons, or rural populations
Social disadvantage	Unfavorable social, economic, or political conditions that some groups of people experience based on their relative position in social hierarchies
Patient navigator	A person who helps guide patients through the healthcare system, including screening, diagnosis, treatment, and follow-up
Carcinogen	Any cancer-causing agent
Genetic	Inherited; having to do with information that is passed from parents to offspring though genes in sperm and egg cells
Genetic risk	Risk factors transmitted at birth through genes
Incidence	Number of newly diagnosed cases during a specific time period
Mortality	Number of deaths during a specific time period
Risk factor	Something that increases the likelihood of developing a disease

(NIH, n.d.; Susan G. Komen Breast Cancer Foundation, Inc., 2019)

What's Known and Unknown About Cancer Among Women of Color?

Cancer and health disparities are well known to be linked to socioeconomic status (SES) and race. They have been observed in relation to specific cancers. For instance, there is a higher incidence of the triple-negative subtype of breast cancer among African American women than women of other racial/ethnic groups, and there are higher rates of cervical cancer incidence and death among Hispanic and African American women than women of other racial/ethnic groups (DeSantis et al., 2019; Agency for Healthcare Research and Quality, n.d.; NIH, 2018).

Lung, breast, colorectal, and cervical cancers are common among low-income women of color. Biological factors may account for some differences, but social factors have a greater influence on these disparities.

Low-income women of color are typically underrepresented in clinical trials (Duma et al., 2018; NIH, 2018; Pasick et al., 2016). Continuing work is needed to identify tailored and effective interventions, while also evaluating the impact of interventions.

Types of Cancer

About 80% of *lung cancer* deaths are thought to be due to smoking; however, people who do not smoke also can have lung cancer. There are a variety of types of lung cancer, with different treatment options and outlooks for each. These include non-small cell lung cancer, which accounts for about 85% of lung cancers; small cell lung cancer, which makes up 10% to 15% of lung cancers; and lung carcinoid tumors, which make up fewer than 5% of lung cancers (American Cancer Society [ACS], 2019b).

Excluding skin cancers, *breast cancer* is the most common cancer type among women. "Breast cancer starts when cells in the breast begin to grow out of control. These cells usually form a tumor that can often be seen on an x-ray or felt as a lump. The tumor is malignant (cancer) if the cells can grow into (invade) surrounding tissues or spread (metastasize) to distant areas of the body. Breast cancer occurs almost entirely in women, but men can get breast cancer, too" (ACS, 2017c).

Colorectal cancer starts in the colon or the rectum. These cancers are named based on where their initial site is. Because they have many features in common, these cancers are usually grouped together (ACS, 2019c).

Cervical cancer "starts in the cells lining the cervix—the lower part of the uterus (womb). This is sometimes called the uterine cervix. The fetus grows in the body of the uterus (the upper part). The cervix connects the body of the uterus to the vagina (birth canal)" (ACS, 2019d). Almost all cases of cervical cancer are caused by (human papillomavirus [HPV]), although not everyone who has had HPV will necessarily get cervical cancer. While rates of cervical cancer have dropped in the U.S. population overall, there is a higher incidence and mortality from cervical cancer in women of color. African American women are twice as likely as White women to die from cervical cancer due to factors such as later stage of cancer at diagnosis, limited access to care, and less aggressive treatment (Arvizo & Mahdi, 2017; Centers for Disease Control and Prevention [CDC], 2018a).

Table I.3 provides information about cancer prevention.

Causes of Cancer and Risk Factors

Lung cancer results from cells in the lung mutating or changing (American Lung Association, 2018). Smoking is the leading cause of lung cancer, causing an estimated 80% to 90% of cases. Current smokers are most at risk, but former smokers, as well as nonsmokers exposed to secondhand smoke, also are at risk of developing lung cancer. Other risk factors include radon exposure, exposure to hazardous chemicals, particle pollution, and genetic risk. These additional risk factors can interact with smoking to further increase risk (American Lung Association, 2018).

Breast cancer is caused by abnormal growth of breast cells; cancerous cells divide more rapidly than healthy cells and continue to grow, causing the formation of a lump or mass. This is likely caused by an interaction of environmental and genetic factors. Certain hormonal, lifestyle, and environmental factors can increase the risk of developing breast cancer. Unfortunately, many of the risk factors, including advancing age and family history of breast cancer, are beyond a patient's control. Being overweight or obese is a risk factor that patients may be able to control, along with other factors such as physical activity and alcohol intake (Mayo Clinic, 2019).

The exact causes of *colorectal cancer* are unknown. Researchers have identified certain risk factors, but the exact relationship between these risk factors and the development of colorectal cancer is yet unidentified. Many lifestyle-related factors have been identified,

Table I.3 What Can Be Done to Prevent Cancer?

	Risk Factors	Behaviors to Reduce Risk	Screening & Early Detection Methods
Lung cancer	• Cigarettes • Cigars and pipes • Environmental tobacco • Smoke (second-hand smoke) • Exposure to: • Radon • Asbestos • Pollution • Lung disease such as tuberculosis	• Do not smoke. • Asbestos workers should use protective equipment. • Avoid radon exposure.	Low-dose computed tomography (LDCT): • Adults aged 55 to 80 years who have a 30 pack-year smoking history and currently smoke or have quit within the past 15 years. • Screening should be discontinued once a person has not smoked for 15 years or develops a health problem that substantially limits life expectancy or the ability or willingness to have curative lung surgery.
Breast cancer	• Family history • Certain breast changes, such as atypical hyperplasia or Lobular carcinoma in situ (LCIS) • Genetic factors • Menopause hormone therapy • Late childbearing • Breast density • Radiation therapy • Alcohol • Over age 60	• Regular exercise • Some evidence suggests a link between diet and breast cancer. • Maintain a healthy weight. • Limit alcohol consumption. • Consult with health provider regarding menopausal hormone use.	• Mammography • Biopsy
Colorectal cancer	• Age (over 55 years) • Diet: seems to be associated with diets high in fat and calories and low in fiber • Polyps: some types of polyps increase risk • Personal medical history • Family medical history • Ulcerative colitis	• Diets low in fat and high in fiber • Regular exercise • Maintain healthy weight. • Limit alcohol consumption. • Polyp removal	• Fecal occult blood test • Digital rectal exam • Sigmoidoscopy • Colonoscopy • Polypectomy • X-rays • Biopsy
Cervical cancer	• Smoking • Early first intercourse • Multiple sexual partners • Sexually transmitted viruses • HPV (causal) • Women whose mothers used synthetic estrogen diethylstilbestrol (DES) during pregnancy	• Limit number of sexual partners. • Safe sex practices • Early detection and treatment for Sexually Transmitted Diseases • Early detection and treatment of precancerous tissue • Stop smoking.	• Pap smear/test • Biopsy

including being overweight or obese; physical inactivity; diets high in red meat or meats cooked at high temperatures; smoking; and heavy alcohol use. Other risk factors, such as older age, a personal history of colorectal polyps or colorectal cancer, a personal history of inflammatory bowel disease, a family history of colorectal cancers, or having an inherited syndrome, are beyond the patient's control (ACS, 2018b). In the United States, African Americans of both sexes are at higher risk for colorectal cancer, although the reasons for this are not completely understood. Further research regarding the causes of these disparities and effective interventions is necessary. Factors such as lack of knowledge of family history, obstacles to accessing care, impact of migration, and lack of clinical data have been identified as contributing to racial disparities in the incidence of colorectal cancer (Jackson et al., 2016).

For *cervical cancer*, HPV infection is the most important, but not the only risk factor. Other important risk factors include smoking, having a weakened immune system, having a chlamydia infection, or being overweight. Additional risk factors include long-term use of oral contraceptives, a diet low in fruits and vegetables, having multiple full-term pregnancies, being younger than 17 at one's first full-term pregnancy, a family history of cervical cancer, and exposure to diethylstilbestrol (DES). Lower SES complicates these other risk factors as it may prevent women from accessing adequate healthcare, including the preventive screenings important for detecting cervical cancer (cervical cancer can be prevented and detected with the HPV vaccine and regular Papanicolaou [Pap] screenings) (ACS, 2017b). Cancers can be caused by DNA mutations that "turn on" *oncogenes* (genes that help cells grow, divide, and stay alive) and turn off *tumor suppressor genes* (genes that keep cell growth under control or make cells die at the right time). Types of HPV cause the production of two proteins that turn off tumor suppressor genes, allowing cells in the cervical lining to grow excessively and develop changes in other genes. In some cases this leads to cancer.

Screening Recommendations

Table I.4 provides screening recommendations based on the type of cancer.

Lung Cancer
The only recommended screening test for lung cancer is low-dose computed tomography (LDCT), a test in which an X-ray machine scans the patient's body and makes detailed images of the lungs using low doses of radiation. A yearly LDCT is recommended for people who (1) have a history of heavy smoking; *and* (2) currently smoke or have quit within the past 15 years; *and* (3) are between 55 and 80 years old. This yearly screening is recommended even in the absence of symptoms; it is the presence of relevant risk factors that determines whether someone needs screening (CDC, 2018b) (Figure I.1).

To determine whether a patient's tobacco use is considered "heavy," a unit known as a "pack-year" is used. A "pack-year" means smoking an average of one pack of cigarettes per day for one year. Thus, someone who has smoked one pack a day for 30 years has a 30 pack-year history and someone who has smoked an average of two packs a day for 15 years also has a 30 pack-year history (CDC, 2018b). Heavy smoking is considered to be a smoking history of 30 or more pack-years. Pack-year calculators such as one available on shouldiscreen.com (University of Michigan, 2019) can help patients determine whether they meet the criterion of heavy use.

Table I.4 ACS Screening Recommendations for Average-Risk, Asymptomatic Adults

Cancer Site	Population	Recommended Screening
Lung	Current or former smokers, ages 55–74	Low-dose helical CT (annually, adults in good health with a 30 pack-year smoking history)
Breast	Women 40–54 years	Mammography (begin regular screening at age 45 or younger, with opportunity to begin annual screenings at 40)
	Women 55 years or older	Mammography (screening every other year, or optional annual screening; continue as long as in good health or have life expectancy of 10 or more years)
Cervix	Women 21–29 years	Pap test (every 3 years)
	Women 30–65 years	Pap test and HPV DNA test (every 3 years with Pap test alone; every 5 years with both tests)
	Women 66 years and older	Pap test and HPV DNA test (may stop cervical cancer screenings if in the last 5 years have had 3 or more consecutive negative Pap tests or 2 or more consecutive combined Pap and HPV DNA tests) * Women who have had a total hysterectomy should stop cervical cancer screening.
Colorectal	Women and men, 45–75 years	Fecal occult blood test; fecal immunochemical test; multi-target stool DNA test; colonoscopy; CT colonoscopy; flexible sigmoidoscopy *Men and women aged 76–85 should make decisions about whether to continue screenings with their doctor. Individuals older than 85 years should be discouraged from continued screening.

Based on information gathered from Smith et al., 2019.

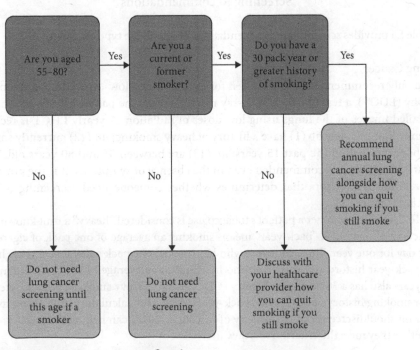

Figure I.1 Lung cancer screening flowchart.

Breast Cancer

Women with an average risk of breast cancer (no personal history or strong family history of breast cancer, no genetic mutation known to increase risk, no chest radiation therapy before age 30) should begin screenings by the age of 45. Between the ages of 40 and 44, a yearly mammogram screening is optional. From ages 45 to 54, however, women should receive regular yearly mammograms. At 55 and older, women can decrease from yearly screenings to a mammogram every other year, or they can choose to continue with yearly mammograms. The ACS recommends that a woman continue screenings as long as she is in good health and is expected to live 10 or more years (Figure I.2).

Recommendations regarding physical breast examinations have recently changed because there is little evidence to show that physical examinations, both those performed by a clinical provider and self-exams, actually help detect breast cancer when women also receive regular mammograms. However, the ACS notes that women should still maintain an awareness of how their breasts usually look and feel and should immediately report any changes to a healthcare provider.

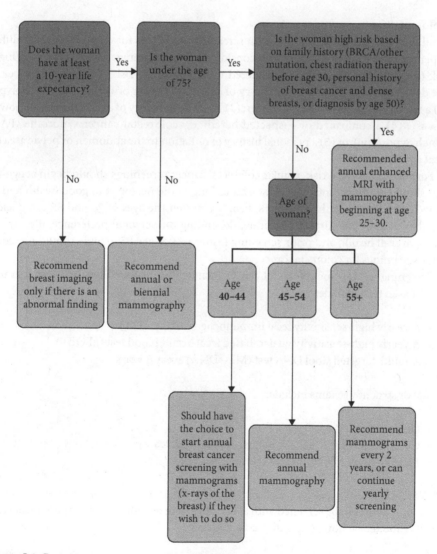

Figure I.2 Breast cancer screening flowchart.

Different guidelines exist for women with a high risk. Women may be classified as high risk for breast cancer if they (1) have a lifetime risk of breast cancer of about 20% to 25% or greater, according to risk assessments based mainly on family history; *or* (2) have a known *BRCA1* or *BRCA2* gene mutation (determined by genetic testing); *or* (3) have a first-degree relative with a *BRCA1* or *BRCA2* gene mutation and have not had genetic testing themselves; *or* (4) had radiation therapy to the chest between the ages of 10 and 30; *or* (5) have Li-Fraumeni syndrome, Cowden syndrome, or Bannayan-Riley-Ruvalcaba syndrome, or have first-degree relatives with any of these syndromes.

Women who meet these criteria and therefore qualify as "high risk" should receive both magnetic resonance imaging (MRI) and a mammogram every year, usually beginning at age 30. MRI screenings are not recommended for women whose lifetime risk of breast cancer is less than 15%. Moreover, when MRI screening is used, it should be in addition to a mammogram rather than on its own. While an MRI is more likely to detect the presence of cancer than a mammogram, it still might miss some cancers that only a mammogram would identify (ACS, 2017a).

Colorectal Cancer

Similar to guidelines for breast cancer, screening guidelines for colorectal cancer differ depending on whether the person is considered to be at average risk or increased/high risk (Figure I.3). A woman is considered to be at average risk of colorectal cancer if she does not have (1) a personal history of colorectal cancer or certain types of polyps; (2) a family history of colorectal cancer; (3) a personal history of an inflammatory bowel disease; (4) a confirmed or suspected hereditary colorectal cancer syndrome (FAP, Lynch Syndrome); or (5) a personal history of radiation to the abdomen or pelvic area to treat a prior cancer.

For those at average risk, regular colorectal cancer screenings should begin at age 45 and should continue until age 75, at least as long as the person is in good health and is expected to live more than 10 years. People between the ages of 76 and 85 can decide whether to continue further screening, depending on personal preference, life expectancy, overall health, and prior screening history. After age 85, people should not continue screenings for colorectal cancer.

Screening options for colorectal cancer include a stool-based test or a visual exam. Stool-based tests include:

- A yearly high-sensitivity fecal immunochemical test (FIT)
- A yearly high-sensitivity guaiac-based fecal occult blood test (gFOBT)
- A multi-targeted stool DNA test (MT-sDNA) every 3 years.

Visual or structural exams include:

- Colonoscopy every 10 years
- CT colonography (virtual colonoscopy) every 5 years
- Flexible sigmoidoscopy (FSIG) every 5 years.

Whichever test is chosen, just getting screened is the most important matter. If someone chooses to be screened with a test other than a colonoscopy, any abnormal test results should be followed up with a colonoscopy.

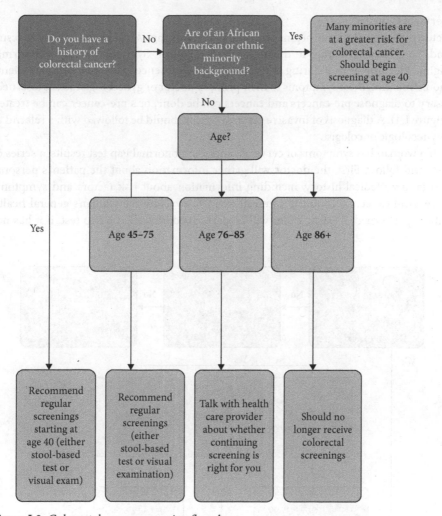

Figure I.3 Colorectal cancer screening flowchart.

People with an increased or high risk of colorectal cancer may need to begin screenings before the age of 45, receive screenings more frequently, and/or get specific tests. People are considered to be at an increased or high risk of colorectal cancer if they (1) have a strong family history of colorectal cancer or certain types of polyps; (2) have a personal history of colorectal cancer of certain types of polyps; (3) have a personal history of inflammatory bowel disease; (4) have a known family history of a hereditary colorectal cancer syndrome (FAP, Lynch syndrome); or (5) have a personal history of radiation to the abdomen or pelvic area to treat a prior cancer. The ACS does not have specific screening guidelines for people at increased or high risk of colorectal cancer. However, other groups, such as the U.S. Multi-Society Task Force on Colorectal Cancer, have issued guidelines, which generally divide people into groups depending on their specific risk factors. These guidelines can be complicated. It is best for healthcare providers to look at these guidelines along with patients to help navigate potentially confusing information (ACS, 2018a).

Cervical Cancer

Detecting cervical cancer begins with the Pap screening. An abnormal Pap test result leads to additional testing to diagnose cervical cancer. Symptoms such as abnormal vaginal bleeding or pain during sex may signal the presence of cervical cancer. Patients should mention these symptoms to their primary doctor or gynecologist so the tests necessary to diagnose pre-cancers and cancers can be done, or a pre-cancer can be treated (Figure I.4). A diagnosis of invasive cervical cancer should be followed with a referral to a gynecologic oncologist.

If a woman has symptoms of cervical cancer, or abnormal Pap test results, a series of tests will follow. First, the doctor will gather information about the patient's personal and family medical history, including information about risk factors and symptoms of cervical cancer. A complete physical exam to evaluate the woman's general health will be performed. A pelvic exam will be performed, as well as a Pap test, if it has not

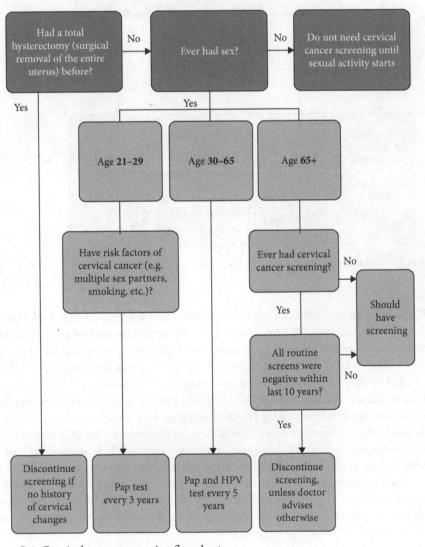

Figure I.4 Cervical cancer screening flowchart.

Table I.5 Cancer Knowledge Posttest

1.	**T**	F	The most common types of cancer among low-income women of color are breast, cervical, colorectal, lung. **Explanation:** Breast, lung, and colorectal cancer are highest in all populations overall. Low-income women and/or women of color are especially at risk for cervical cancer.
2.	**T**	F	Breast cancer is the leading cause of cancer for women, except for skin cancers. **Explanation:** About one in eight women will develop breast cancer. It is the second leading cause of cancer death for women, following lung cancer. While lung cancer is more fatal, breast cancer is more common in women.
3.	**T**	F	Detecting cervical cancer begins with the Pap screening. **Explanation:** The Pap screening is the first line of testing to detect the presence of cervical cancer. Further diagnostic tests follow the Pap screening to actually diagnose the presence of cervical cancer.
4.	T	**F**	There is nothing that can be done to prevent cancer. **Explanation:** Various measures can be taken to help prevent cancer or detect it early. These may include lifestyle factors such as avoiding smoking, improving one's diet, exercising, using sunscreen, or other measures. Regular screening also can help to detect the presence of cancer early.
5.	**T**	F	Smoking is the leading cause of lung cancer. **Explanation:** About 80% of cancer deaths are thought to result from smoking, although not everyone who smokes will develop lung cancer, and people who don't smoke can develop lung cancer.

been performed already. The patient's lymph nodes will be felt to check for evidence of metastasis—that is, cancer spread (ACS, 2016).

The Pap test is a screening test rather than a diagnostic test. To diagnose cervical cancer, other tests are necessary. These tests include colposcopy (with biopsy), endocervical scraping, and cone biopsies. The colposcopy follows an abnormal Pap result or the presence of symptoms suggestive of cervical cancer. The colposcopy is performed as a pelvic exam, using a speculum and a magnifying instrument called a colposcope. A biopsy may be ordered if abnormalities are identified.

References

Agency for Healthcare Research and Quality. (n.d.). 2018 national healthcare quality and disparities report. AHRQ. https://www.ahrq.gov/research/findings/nhqrdr/nhqdr18/index.html

American Cancer Society. (2016). Tests for cervical cancer. https://www.cancer.org/cancer/cervical-cancer/detection-diagnosis-staging/how-diagnosed.html

American Cancer Society. (2017a). American Cancer Society recommendations for the early detection of breast cancer. https://www.cancer.org/cancer/breastcancer/screening-tests-and-early-detection/american-cancer-society-recommendations-for-the-early-detection-of-breast-cancer.html

American Cancer Society. (2017b). Do we know what causes cervical cancer? https://www.cancer.org/cancer/cervical-cancer/causes-risks-prevention/what-causes.html

American Cancer Society. (2017c). What is breast cancer? https://www.cancer.org/cancer/breast-cancer/about/what-is-breast-cancer.html

American Cancer Society. (2018a). American Cancer Society guideline for colorectal cancer screening. https://www.cancer.org/cancer/colon-rectal-cancer/detection-diagnosis-staging/acs-recommendations.html

American Cancer Society. (2018b). What causes colorectal cancer? https://www.cancer.org/cancer/colon-rectal-cancer/causes-risks-prevention/whatcauses.html

American Cancer Society. (2019a). Cancer facts for women. https://www.cancer.org/healthy/find-cancer-early/womens-health/cancer-facts-for-women.html

American Cancer Society. (2019b). Lung cancer. https://www.cancer.org/cancer/lung-cancer.html

American Cancer Society. (2019c). What is colorectal cancer? https://www.cancer.org/cancer/colon-rectal-cancer/about/what-is-colorectal-cancer.html

American Cancer Society. (2019d). What is cervical cancer? https://www.cancer.org/cancer/cervical-cancer/about/what-is-cervical-cancer.html

American Cancer Society. (2019e). Cancer facts & figures 2019. https://www.cancer.org/content/dam/cancer-org/research/cancer-facts-and-statistics/annual-cancer-facts-and-figures/2019/cancer-facts-and-figures-2019.pdf

American Lung Association. (2018). What causes lung cancer. https://www.lung.org/lung-health-and-diseases/lung-disease-lookup/lung-cancer/learn-about-lung-cancer/what-is-lung-cancer/what-causes-lung-cancer.html

Arvizo, C., & Mahdi, H. (2017). Disparities in cervical cancer in African American women: What primary care physicians can do. *Cleveland Clinic Journal of Medicine*, *84*(10), 788–794. https://www.mdedge.com/ccjm/article/147719/oncology/disparities-cervical-cancer-african-american-women-what-primary-care

Centers for Disease Control and Prevention. (2018). HPV-associated cancers rates by race and ethnicity. https://www.cdc.gov/cancer/hpv/statistics/race.htm

Centers for Disease Control and Prevention. (2018). Who should be screened for lung cancer? https://www.cdc.gov/cancer/lung/basic_info/screening.htm

DeSantis, C. E., Ma, J., Gaudet, M. M., Newman, L. A., Miller, K. D., Goding Sauer, A., Jemal, A., & Siegel, R. L. (2019). Breast cancer statistics, 2019. *CA: A Cancer Journal for Clinicians*, *69*(6), 438–451. https://doi.org/10.3322/caac.21583

Duma, N., Vera Aguilera, J., Paludo, J., Haddox, C. L., Gonzalez Velez, M., Wang, Y., Leventakos, K., Hubbard, J. M., Mansfield, A. S., Go, R. S., & Adjei, A. A. (2018). Representation of minorities and women in ONCOLOGY clinical Trials: Review of the past 14 years. *Journal of Oncology Practice*, *14*(1). https://doi.org/10.1200/jop.2017.025288

Jackson, C. S., Oman, M., Patel, A. M., & Vega, K. J. (2016). Health disparities in colorectal cancer among racial and ethnic minorities in the United States. *Journal of Gastrointestinal Oncology*, *7*(Suppl. 1), S32–S43. doi:10.3978/j.issn.2078-6891.2015.039

Mayo Clinic. (2019). Breast cancer. https://www.mayoclinic.org/diseasesconditions/breast-cancer/symptoms-causes/syc-20352470

National Cancer Institute. (2018). Cancer health disparities research. https://www.cancer.gov/research/areas/disparities

National Cancer Institute. (2019). Cancer disparities. https://www.cancer.gov/about-cancer/understanding/disparities

National Cancer Institute. (n.d.) NCI dictionary of cancer terms: Patient navigator. https://www.cancer.gov/publications/dictionaries/cancer-terms/def/patient-navigator

Pasick, R. J., Joseph, G., Stewart, S., Kaplan, C., Lee, R., Luce, J., Davis, S., Marquez, T., Nguyen, T., & Guerra, C. (2016). Effective Referral of Low-Income Women at Risk for Hereditary Breast and Ovarian Cancer to Genetic Counseling: A Randomized Delayed Intervention Control Trial. *American Journal of Public Health*, *106*(10), 1842–1848. https://doi.org/10.2105/AJPH.2016.303312

Smith, R. A., Andrews, K. S., Brooks, D., Fedewa, S. A., Manassaram-Baptiste, D., Saslow, D., & Wender, R. C. (2019). Cancer screening in the United States, 2019: A review of current American Cancer Society guidelines and current issues in cancer screening. *CA Cancer Journal for Clinicians, 69*(3), 184–210.

Susan G. Komen Breast Cancer Foundation, Inc. (2019). Komen perspectives: Breast cancer disparities. https://blog.komen.org/blog/komen-perspectives-breast-cancer-disparities/

University of Michigan. (2019). Pack-year calculator. https://shouldiscreen.com/English/pack-year-calculator

Module I.2: Chronic Care Conceptual Model

At the heart of cancer prevention is the belief that an empowered patient will reject cancer fatalism and will demand partnership of her care with her provider. As the locus of control shifts toward the patient, there are greater opportunities for chronic disease self-management, with better cancer outcomes related to improved quality of life (Brincks et al., 2010). Certain tools and strategies, including use of behavioral theories such as social cognitive theory, are particularly adaptable to help low-income women increase their awareness and adoption of cancer interventions. Social cognitive theory, which is based on the constructs of self-efficacy, environment, behavioral capability, expectations, expectancies, self-control and performance, observational learning, and reinforcement, have been demonstrated to increase embrace of physical exercise among patients with breast cancer, which improves perceived quality of life (Rogers et al., 2004). However, a limitation of behavioral health theories such as social cognitive theory and stages of change is that they do not permit a full contextualization of a patient's illness, including her ability to access a provider, navigate a complex healthcare system, and secure the resources needed to manage her underlying chronic disease.

The chronic care model (CCM) has emerged as one of several multi-level strategies that can be adapted for chronic disease management, particularly cancer prevention and management for low-income women (Barr et al., 2003). This conceptual model acknowledges the social and structural determinants of health and encourages proactive approaches for improving health by integrating care at the community, organizational, practice, and patient level. By creating partnerships between health systems and communities, the patient is "activated" to become the prime mover of resources needed to promote chronic disease self-management (Figure I.5).

The CCM is a critical component of the Health Disparities Collaboratives, which were developed by the Bureau of Primary Health Care (BPHC) in order to improve overall healthcare and to eliminate health disparities (Chin, 2010). BPHC, a part of the U.S. Department of Health and Human Services, is responsible for funding programs to expand access to high-quality, culturally and linguistically competent, primary and preventive care for underserved, uninsured, and underinsured Americans. The Health

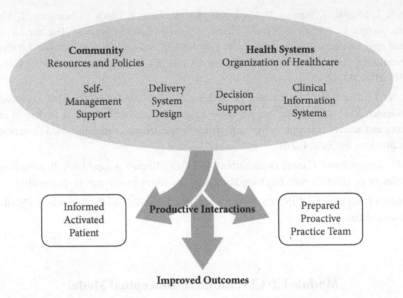

Figure I.5 The chronic care model.

Disparities Collaboratives strive to achieve excellence in practice and promote health equity through the following goals:

- Generate and document improved health outcomes for underserved populations
- Transform clinical practice through models of care, improvement, and learning
- Develop infrastructure, expertise, and multidisciplinary leadership to support and drive improved health status
- Build strategic partnerships.

The Health Disparities Cancer Collaboratives (HDCC) arose from the Health Disparities Collaboratives as a quality improvement program designed to increase the cancer control activities of screening and follow-up among underserved populations. The HDCCs were operational among community health centers supported by the Health Resources and Services Administration (HRSA) to serve financially, functionally, and culturally vulnerable populations (Harmon & Carlson, 1991).

To effect fundamental changes in the healthcare delivery systems needed to eliminate health disparities, the Health Disparities Collaboratives urged adherence to the CCM. The CCM was developed by a national program of the Robert Wood Johnson Foundation, called Improving Chronic Illness Care, at the MacColl Center for Health Care Innovation in Seattle, Washington (Wagner, 1998). By the 1990s the CCM was one of the most popular conceptual frameworks for teaching and implementing chronic disease management. It is estimated that by 2030, 171 million people will require chronic disease management (Anderson, 2010; Wu & Green, 2000). Consequently, there is heightened interest in developing a conceptual framework such as the CCM that mitigates the deficiencies in our current management of chronic diseases. The CCM consists of six components of healthcare delivery (Table I.6):

Table I.6 Chronic Care Model (CCM) Components

Model Components		Examples
Health system— Organization of healthcare	Program planning that includes measuring goals for better care of chronic illness	• Visible support of improvements provided by senior leadership
Self-management support	Emphasis on the importance of the central role that patients have in managing their own care	• Educational resources, skills training, and psychosocial support provided to patients to assist them in managing their care
Decision support	Integration of evidence-based guidelines into daily clinical practice	• Wide dissemination of practice guidelines • Education and specialist support provided to healthcare team
Delivery system design	Focus on teamwork and an expanded scope of practice for team members to support chronic care	• Planned visits and sustained follow-up • Clearly define roles of healthcare team
Clinical information systems	Developing information systems based on patient populations to provide relevant client data	• Surveillance system that provides alert, recall, and follow-up information • Identification of relevant patient subgroups requiring proactive care
Community resources and policies	Developing partnerships with community organizations that support and meet patients' needs	• Identify effective programs and encourage appropriate participation • Referral to relevant community-based services

(Wagner, 1999)

1. Health System/Organizational Support—Create a culture, organization, and mechanisms that promote safe, high-quality care.
   a. Visibly support improvement at all levels, beginning with leadership. Promote effective improvement strategies designed for comprehensive system change.
   b. Encourage open and systematic handling of errors and quality problems to improve care.
   c. Provide incentives based on quality of care.
   d. Develop agreements that support care coordination within and across organizations.
2. Clinical Information Systems—Organize patient and population data to facilitate efficient and effective care.
   a. Provide timely reminders for providers and patients.
   b. Identify relevant subpopulations for proactive care.
   c. Facilitate individual patient care planning.
   d. Share information with patients and providers to coordinate care.
   e. Monitor performance of practice team and care system.
3. Delivery System Design—Assure the delivery of effective, efficient clinical care and self-management support.
   a. Define roles and distribute tasks among team members.
   b. Use planned interactions to support evidence-based care.
   c. Provide clinical case management services for complex patients.

    d. Ensure regular follow-up by the care team.

    e. Give care that patients understand and that fits with their cultural background.

4. Decision Support—Promote clinical care that is consistent with scientific evidence and patient preferences.

    a. Embed evidence-based guidelines into daily clinical practice.

    b. Share evidence-based guidelines and information with patients to encourage their participation.

    c. Use proven provider education methods.

    d. Integrate specialist expertise and primary care.

5. Self-Management Support—Empower and prepare patients to manage their health and health care.

    a. Emphasize the patient's central role in managing their health.

    b. Use effective self-management support strategies that include assessment, goal-setting, action planning, problem-solving, and follow-up.

    c. Organize internal and community resources to provide ongoing self-management support to patients.

6. Community Resources—Mobilize community resources to meet needs of patients.

    a. Encourage patients to participate in effective community programs.

    b. Form partnerships with community organizations to support and develop interventions that fill gaps in needed services.

    c. Advocate for policies to improve patient care.

Improved outcomes accrue when enhanced intersectionality of the model's six components leads to a prepared, proactive practice team and an informed, activated patient. There is now significant evidence that the CCM is effective in both chronic care management and in practice improvement (Davy et al., 2015).

David Haggstrom, along with colleagues at Indiana University and the National Cancer Institute, explored whether Health Disparities Cancer Collaboratives that implemented the CCM were more likely to increase cancer screening and follow-up among underserved populations from 2003 to 2005 (Haggstrom et al., 2012). In this study, community health centers were recruited from two groups: a collaborative group (19 centers) that had participated in the HDCC and a matched control group (21 centers) that did not participate in the collaborative (Figure I.6). Eighty-six percent (19/22) of health centers that participated in the HDCC were recruited into this study. A matched control health center was selected for each HDCC center based upon region, urban/rural designation, and number of patients.

CCM implementation was measured for the six components of the model (Wagner, 1999), comprising the following a priori subscales, each consisting of two survey items:

1. Self-management support (goal-setting, shared decision-making)
2. Clinical decision support (patient education, provider reminders)
3. Delivery system design (role redesign, appointment redesign)
4. Clinical information systems (performance feedback for providers and teams)
5. Healthcare organization (leadership expectations and recognition)
6. Community resources (measured with a single item).

Cancer care process improvement was measured through self-report in the organizational surveys.

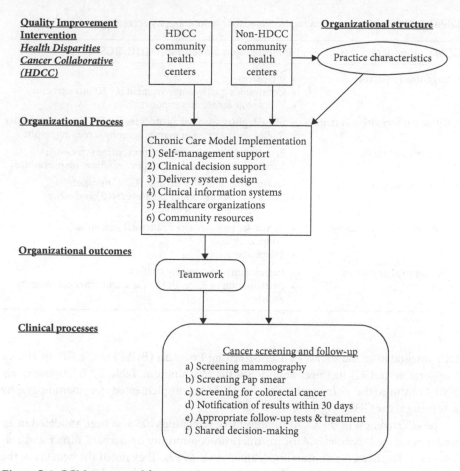

Figure I.6 CCM conceptual framework.

Overall, CCM implementation was significantly more likely among health centers that participated in the collaborative than centers that did not. There were also significant differences in the implementation of self-management support, clinical decision support, delivery system design, and clinical information systems. CCM implementation was independently associated with cancer care process improvement.

The CCM posits that perverse incentives in our U.S. healthcare system drive poor clinical outcomes, and that realignment of healthcare systems with a focus on patient-centered care can improve outcomes for patients living with chronic conditions. There is reason to believe that reengineering our healthcare system can also lead to effective preventive care and that the CCM can be modified to a more utilitarian "care model" for preventive care. Although there are differences between preventive care and management of existing chronic illnesses, there are far more similarities (Glasgow et al., 2001). There is a great deal of overlap in the healthcare system changes and characteristics required to deliver quality preventive and chronic illness care.

The CCM appears congruent with other frameworks for conceptualizing prevention activities (Dickey et al., 1999; Goldstein & DePue, 1998; Solberg et al., 1997) and consistent with clinical experience and the empirical literature on preventive interventions, as illustrated by the following example of breast cancer screening. The CCM is

Table I.7 CCM Components as Implemented for Mammography Screenings at GHC

CCM Component	Mammography Screening at GHC: BCSP
1. Organization of care	• Incentives • Continuous quality improvement (CQI) infrastructure • Visible top-leadership support
2. Clinical information systems	• BCSP registry with risk profiles for women aged 40 and older • Radiology database of mammography screening results
3. Delivery system design	• Proactive written invitations for routine screening; personal contact for those requiring follow-up procedures
4. Decision support	• Online tools available through GHC intranet • National Cancer Center Institute (NCI) and other evidence-based guidelines
5. Self-management support	• Reminder postcards and outreach scheduling class for nonparticipants • Telephone counseling
6. Community resources	• Regional mammography centers • Participation in Race for the Cure and other community events

fully integrated in the Breast Cancer Screening Program (BCSP) at the Group Health Cooperative (GHC) in Puget Sound, Seattle, Washington. Table I.7 (Glasgow et al., 2001) outlines the components of the CCM as implemented for mammography screening at the GHC.

The effectiveness of the CCM in preventive screenings has also been validated in an under-resourced, primarily African American community by Barbara Rimer and colleagues in Durham, North Carolina (Rimer et al., 1999). They noted the benefits of the CCM in promoting cancer screenings, including mammography and Pap testing, among 1,318 low-income African American women. Operationalized components of the CCM included clinical information systems, which included individualized print materials, self-management support through printouts of recommended screening intervals, and system-generated phone prompts. The combined phone, print, and prompting interventions were particularly effective in enhancing Pap test compliance, achieving 70% compliance for some women without hysterectomies.

A new model integrating chronic care with population health and behavioral health theory, developed by Victoria Barr and colleagues (Barr et al., 2003) was even bolder and more comprehensive than the earlier model. The expanded CCM (Figure I.7) both acknowledges and operationalizes the role of the social determinants of health in influencing individual, community, and population health (Barr et al., 2003). In the expanded CCM, the border between the health system and the community is porous, representing a seamless flow of ideas, resources, and people. The four critical areas within the health system—self-management support, decision support, delivery system design, and information systems—are more contiguous with the community line, illustrating a stronger integration. Three key community principles—build healthy public policy, create supportive environments, and strengthen community action—are explicitly outlined. The net effect is a model that more precisely merges with population health promotion.

Even with the fidelity of the CCM and its use in cancer prevention and management, there is a lack of clarity about the concept of chronic care coordination and an uncertainty

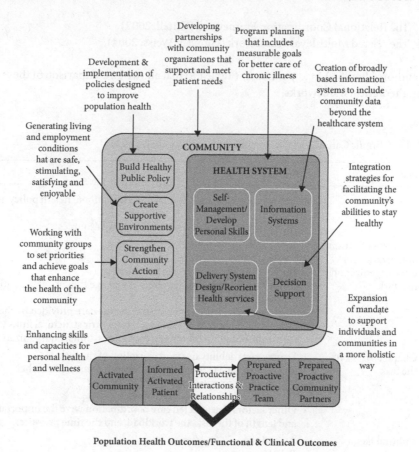

Figure I.7 Expanded CCM: Integrating Population Health. Reprinted with permission, Virginia Barr et al. 2003, Hospital Quarterly, 7(1), 73–82.

on how to evaluate interventions. This is partly related to a need for a uniform definition of care coordination. A case definition of care coordination was provided in a landmark review conducted by the Agency for Healthcare Research and Quality (Van Houdt et al., 2013):

> The deliberate organization of patient care activities between two or more participants (including the patient) involved in a patient's care to facilitate the appropriate delivery of health care services. Organizing care involves the marshalling of personnel and other resources needed to carry out all required patient care activities and is often managed by the exchange of information among participants responsible for different aspects of care.

In the review, five theoretical frameworks were described to show how theoretical thinking to clarify key concepts could enrich the study of care coordination:

1. The Andersen Behavioral Model (Andersen, 1995)
2. The Donabedian Quality Framework (Donabedian, 1966)
3. The Organizational Design Framework (Nadler & Tushman, 1988), where Wagner's CCM (Wagner, 1998) was described as an example in the landmark review

4. The Relational Coordination Framework (Gittell, 2002)
5. The related Multi-level Framework (Gittell & Weiss, 2004).

The authors identified 14 key concepts (Table I.8) that allowed a comparison of these different theoretical frameworks.

Table I.8 Chronic Care Model (CCM) Concepts and Components

Concepts	Components
1. External factors	• How care coordination was affected by national health policy and economic factors • Dependency on regulations and existing resources
2. Structure of a team, organization, or inter-organizational network	• Number of participants • Specializations • Number of linkages between participants • Amount of information required to manage the care of the patient or patient group • Existing mechanisms for coordinating the care provided by the different participants; for example, leaders or structural links across the boundaries between disciplines, units, or organizations
3. Characteristics of the task	• Degree of variability or standardization of the tasks • Degree to which team members depended upon each other • Simplicity or complexity of the tasks • Degree of certainty in the outcome • Other factors that affected care coordination were the importance and length of the task, the workload, and the time pressure.
4. Cultural factors	• Attitudes • Beliefs • Norms • Values
5. Knowledge and technology	• Available skills • Expertise • Training • Information
6. Need for coordination	• Need to exchange information • Need to provide and coordinate care
7. Administrative operational processes	• Impersonal methods involving standardized arrangements and minimal feedback, like guidelines • Personal methods, involving personal interactions between individual collaborators, or between a team and an assigned coordinator, with a considerable degree of feedback, like a personal contact between healthcare professionals • Group methods, involving joint planning and decision-making with maximum feedback, like team meetings
8. Exchange of information	• Transfer of information, ideas, and opinions among the members of a team, within an organization, or between organizations
9. Goals	• Importance of setting common goals • Sharing these goals • Ensuring collective ownership of these goals
10. Roles	• Definition of roles and the awareness of each other's roles
11. Quality of relationships	• Addressing the quality of relationships promoted mutual respect and high-quality collaboration.

Table I.8 Continued

Concepts	Components
12. Patient outcome	• The patient's perception or the patient's evaluation of healthcare professionals' performance regarding patient health status • Patient satisfaction • Continuity of care • Patient safety, efficiency, efficacy, availability, accessibility, and compatibility
13. Team outcome	• Team behavior and team satisfaction
14. Organizational or inter-organizational outcome	• Comprehensiveness • Accessibility • Compatibility • Conflict • Efficiency of the organization

Frameworks 4 and 5, the Relational Coordination Framework and the Multilevel Framework, addressed the same key concepts. Both advocate the use of the same organizational mechanisms within and between organizations, allowing networks to become more strengthened, which leads to higher quality and greater efficiency of care (Gittell, 2002; Gittell & Weiss, 2004). Only the Andersen Behavioral Model fully addresses cultural factors such as attitudes, beliefs, norms, and values (Andersen, 1995). These cultural factors are essential when engaging in the cross-cultural communications that empower low-income women with cancer to become activated, engaged partners. Improved patient outcomes are the ultimate goal of the CCM and theoretical frameworks discussed above. All five frameworks succeed in improving patient outcomes through care coordination.

Conclusion

The CCM, crafted to drive care coordination and promote chronic disease self-management, has been proven effective as a framework for prevention of chronic diseases. It has at times been called simply "the care model." It has been demonstrated to be a useful template to guide cancer prevention strategies and has been validated in a population of low-income African American women with cancer. However, no one model can be 100% effective and generalizable to all communities. Practitioners and social scientists who seek to reduce health disparities should become familiar with key behavioral theories such as social cognitive theory and stages of change, as well as the five theoretical frameworks for the study of care coordination that are highlighted in this handbook. A new, expanded CCM (see Figure I.7), integrating chronic care with population health and behavioral health theory, is more comprehensive and actionable than the earlier version. Future iterations of the care model should explicitly mention the social and structural barriers to health and should highlight the components associated with population health promotion. Nonetheless, the current care model with the prevention components should be deployed more often in our unwavering efforts to reduce cancer in low-income women.

References

Andersen, G. (2010). Chronic care: Making the case for ongoing care. Robert Wood Johnson Foundation. https://www.rwjf.org/en/library/research/2010/01/chronic-care.html

Andersen, R. M. (1995). Revisiting the behavioral model and access to medical care: Does it matter? *Journal of Health and Social Behavior, 36*(1), 1–10.

Barr, V., Robinson, S., Marin-Link, B., Underhill, L., Dotts, A., Ravensdale, D., & Salivaras, S. (2003). The expanded chronic care model: An integration of concepts and strategies from population health promotion and the chronic care model. *Hospital Quarterly, 7*(1), 73–82.

Brincks, A., Feaster, D., Burns, M., & Behar-Zusman, V. (2010). The influence of health locus of control on the patient-provider relationship. *Psychology, Health & Medicine, 15*, 720–728. doi:10.1080/13548506.2010.498921

Chin, M. H. (2010). Quality improvement implementation and disparities: The case of the Health Disparities Collaboratives. *Medical Care, 48*, 668–675.

Davy, C., Bleasel, J., Liu, H., Tchan, M., Ponniah, S., & Brown, A. (2015). Effectiveness of chronic care models: Opportunities for improving healthcare practice and health outcomes: A systematic review. *BMC Health Services Research, 15*, 194. doi:10.1186/s12913-015-0854-8

Dickey, L. L., Gemson, D. H., & Carney, P. (1999). Office system interactions supporting primary care-based health behavior change counseling. *American Journal of Preventive Medicine, 17*, 299–308.

Donabedian, A. (1966). Evaluating the quality of medical care. *Milbank Memorial Fund Quarterly, 44*(3), Suppl. 206.

Gittell, J. H. (2002). Coordinating mechanisms in care provider groups: Relational coordination as a mediator and input uncertainty as a moderator of performance effects. *Management Science, 48*(11), 1408–1426.

Gittell, J. H., & Weiss, S. J. (2004). Coordination networks within and across organizations: A multilevel framework. *Journal of Management Studies, 41*(1), 127–153.

Glasgow, R. E., Orleans, C. T., & Wagner, E. H. (2001). Does the chronic care model serve also as a template for improving prevention? *Milbank Quarterly, 79*(4), 579–612. doi:10.1111/1468-0009.00222

Goldstein, M. R., & DePue, J. (1998). Models for provider-patient interaction: Applications to health behavior change. In S. Shumaker, E. B. Schron, & W. L. McBee (Eds.), *The handbook of health behavior change*. Springer, 85–113.

Haggstrom, D. A., Taplin, S. H., Monahan, P., & Clauser, S. (2012). Chronic care model implementation for cancer screening and follow-up in community health centers. *Journal of Health Care for the Poor and Underserved, 23*, 49–66.

Harmon, R. G., & Carlson, R. H. (1991). HRSA's role in primary care and public health in the 1990s. *Public Health Reports, 106*(1), 6–10.

Nadler, D, & Tushman, M. (1988). *Strategic organization design*. Scott, Foresman and Company.

Rimer, B. K., Conway, M., Lyna, P., Glassman, B., Yarnall, K. S. H., Lipkus, I., & Barber, L. T. (1999). The impact of tailored interventions on a community health center population. *Patient Education and Counseling, 37*, 125–140.

Rogers, L. Q., Matevey, C., Hopkins-Price, P., Shah, P., Dunnington, G., & Courneya, K. S. (2004). Exploring social cognitive theory constructs for promoting exercise among breast cancer patients. *Cancer Nursing, 27*(6), 462–473. doi:10.1097/00002820-200411000-00006

Solberg, L. I., Kottke, T. E., Conn, S. A., Brekke, M. L., Calomeni, C. A., & Conboy, K. S. (1997). Delivering clinical preventive services is a systems problem. *Annals of Behavioral Medicine, 19,* 271–278.

Van Houdt, S., Heyrman, J., Vanhaecht, K., Sermeus, W., & De Lepeleire, J. (2013). An in-depth analysis of theoretical frameworks for the study of care coordination. *International Journal of Integrated Care, 13*(2). https://www.ijic.org/articles/10.5334/ijic.1068/

Wagner, E. H. (1998). Chronic disease management: What will it take to improve care for chronic illness? *Effective Clinical Practice, 1*(1), 2–4.

Wagner, E. H. (1999). Care of older people with chronic illness. In E. Calkins, C. Boult, & E. H. Wagner (Eds.), *New ways to care for older people: Building systems based on evidence.* Springer, 39–64.

Wu, S-Y., & Green, A. (2000). *Projection of chronic illness prevalence and cost inflation.* RAND Corporation.

1

Interpersonal, Community, and Population Communication and Engagement

> Focus group participant (St. Louis community resident): "I smoked from age 13. Back in the day, you didn't know cigarettes were cancerous. So, I smoked from 13 to 33. And one night, I went to work, and it was kind of drizzling, and I had to jog to Union Station across the street to the post office. I was out of breath. The cigarettes that I had in that pack, I said that when I get through with these I'm not smoking anymore."
>
> Wells et al., 2019

The opening quote in this chapter speaks to the vulnerability and lack of access to basic information of low-income women of color and the dangers posed by everyday health risks. While cigarette smoking is but one risk, this chapter reveals that cancer is a collection of related diseases. Using the chronic care model (CCM) as the overarching theoretical framework, we highlight that while biological factors may account for some differences, social factors, peer pressures, and lack of communication about the "known" and "unknown" facts often have an even greater influence on disparities.

Module 1.1: Cancer Communication

This module provides an overview and examples of how various communication strategies and interventions can be used to support and improve screening and treatment adherence among low-income women. Standards are discussed for community-engaged strategies to facilitate development of plain-language communication and education materials that use visual composition, layout, and design to address and support health literacy. Health literacy tips for navigators and lay and community health workers are provided. Strategies are described to assess barriers and stressors that affect cancer prevention behaviors and treatment adherence frequently encountered by low-income women. Finally, the impact of unique values, beliefs, and cultural practices on health education and behaviors is discussed, with recommendations for application in cancer education and communication.

Communication is key to adherence and health outcomes. Moreover, communication is central to the implementation of the expanded CCM, especially in terms of patient self-management. Effective communication has powerful effects on whether a woman

Cancer Navigation. Anjanette A. Wells, Vetta L. Sanders Thompson, Will Ross, Carol Camp Yeakey, and Sheri R. Notaro, Oxford University Press. © Oxford University Press 2022. DOI: 10.1093/med/9780190672867.003.0002

decides to go in for her routine mammogram screening or keeps her chemotherapy appointment. Communication can also improve health through better continuity of care, patient satisfaction, and a commitment to screening or treatment over a life course (Cabana & Jee, 2004; Fuertes et al., 2007; Vermeir et al., 2015). This can be particularly important for women who have misperceptions about screening or prior negative experiences with systems of care. Effective cancer communication includes many elements. Among low-income women of color, key adherence drivers (O'Toole et al., 2019) include a trusting patient–provider relationship (Committee on Improving the Quality of Cancer Care, 2013), culturally tailored print information (Ka'opua et al., 2011), and adequate health literacy (Benjamin, 2010). In fact, when clinicians are perceived as more informative, caring, and interested in the patient's views, effective communication has the power to decrease perceived social distance and increases patient trust during the consultation (Gordon et al., 2006). In this chapter, we will see how communication can be critical to health outcomes. Additionally, we will discuss health literacy, a modifiable practice that can be targeted for interventions to increase the chances that communication will accomplish desired health outcomes.

Health Literacy: Literacy in Support of Health

Encouraging patient screening and self-management of health takes more than just information exchange. It also comprises patient literacy in support of health, which is health literacy. Health literacy is an important social determinant of health (Kreps, 2006; Lee et al., 2015). Difficulties in communication contribute to unequal access to health information and less patient participation in healthcare decision-making. Ultimately, these factors result in the health disparities observed among low-income women of color (Kreps, 2006).

Health literacy is the ability to obtain, process, and understand the basic health information and services needed to make appropriate health decisions (Centers for Disease Control and Prevention, 2016). This is an important factor in patient–provider relationships with women because it affects their ability to understand clinical and health-related information, thus making truly informed decisions. Poor health literacy might restrict a woman's ability to understand and to be an active participant in meaningful medical appointments. The definition of health literacy from the Patient Protection and Affordable Care Act (ACA) of 2010, Title V is more inclusive. The ACA definition includes an individual's ability to communicate about health information (Centers for Disease Control and Prevention, 2016). In addition, health literacy includes numeracy skills, as health activities include measurements related to the consumption of calories and nutrients, calculations related to energy expenditure and weight management, and measurement of medication and biometrics as a part of disease management. For example, calculating cholesterol and blood sugar levels, measuring medications, and understanding nutrition labels all require math skills. General literacy and numeracy skills are involved in the ability to choose between health plans by reading and comparing coverages, including calculating premiums, copays, and deductibles. According to the National Assessment of Adult Literacy, only 12% of adults have "proficient" health literacy and 14% of adults (30 million people) have "below basic" health literacy (Centers for Disease Control and Prevention, 2016; U.S. Wolf et al., 2007). Adults with "below basic" health literacy are more likely to report that their health is poor compared to adults with "proficient" health literacy (Centers for Disease Control and Prevention, 2016; Wolf et al., 2007).

Healthcare organizations can help address literacy-related barriers by providing patients with culturally appropriate health education that helps them to understand their health issues, encourages patient participation in discussing concerns and beliefs, and provides suggestions for how to talk with their physicians (Glanz et al., 2008; Jongen et al., 2018). Title VI and the Department of Health and Human Services regulations require all entities receiving federal financial assistance, including healthcare organizations, to take steps to ensure that individuals with limited English proficiency (LEP) have meaningful access to the services they provide (Limited English Proficiency, 2021). Individuals who do not speak English as their primary language and who have a limited ability to read, write, speak, or understand English may be considered to have LEP and may be eligible to receive language assistance (Limited English Proficiency, 2021). The key to providing meaningful access for LEP individuals is to ensure that effective communication between the healthcare organization and the patient is readily available. When working with women with LEP, it is important not to make assumptions about the best ways to communicate with them. Similarly, in many cultures it is customary to call people by their last names, especially when they are older than you. So, it is important to ask your patients not only their preferred language, but also how they would like to be referred to. It is very important not to assume. For example, some family members may not use American Sign Language to communicate with their deaf or hard-of-hearing family members; the family members might be able to manage only a few uncomplicated communication tasks in a straightforward manner (Ohio Mental Health and Addiction Services, 2019). Just as important is to be mindful of your verbal and nonverbal communications, as well as your actions. It is too easy to harm someone by not being aware of what is (and is not) respectful and appropriate.

We cannot understand the importance of cultural competence without the inclusion of providing accessible, culturally appropriate oral and written language services to LEP patients through such means as bilingual/bicultural staff, trained medical interpreters, and qualified translators. It is important for individuals and systems to communicate effectively and to convey information in a manner that is easily understood by diverse audiences, including persons with LEP, those who have low literacy skills or are not literate, and individuals with disabilities. This also requires the capacity of organizations to respond effectively to the needs of the populations they serve (Betancourt & Tan-McGrory, 2014; Wilson, 2013). To do so, healthcare organizations must have policies, practices, procedures, and earmarked resources to support that capacity (Betancourt & Tan-McGrory, 2014; Wilson, 2013).

Poor health literacy is a complex issue, with serious individual and social consequences. Health literacy affects people's ability to:

- Navigate the healthcare system, including filling out health and business forms, as well as the ability to obtain services
- Provide accurate health histories
- Engage in cancer and chronic-disease management
- Understand information on probability and risk that is related to decisions about treatment of cancer and other diseases
- Fully participate in health decision-making.

People with limited health literacy may lack knowledge or have mistaken beliefs about the body and the causes of disease, including cancer. Those with health issues may not understand the relationship between health behaviors such as diet and exercise and various health outcomes.

Literacy can be defined as the ability to read, write, speak, and compute and solve problems at levels that permit individuals to maintain employment, engage in civic activities, and continue to develop knowledge and skills necessary for societal and individual well-being. It is fundamental to efforts to improve health literacy. We know that education and language are factors that affect a person's health literacy skills (National Center for Education Statistics, 2006). Low literacy is also linked to poor health outcomes such as higher rates of hospitalization and less frequent use of preventive services (Centers for Disease Control and Prevention, 2016). The ability to improve health literacy may be linked to the problem-solving and life-long learning aspects of literacy. In addition to the basic literacy skills required, health literacy requires knowledge of health topics, which is also dependent on basic literacy skills.

While biological literacy is not often discussed as a part of health literacy, it has particular relevance as advances are made in the understanding of disease biology, genetics, and treatment (Miller, 207). According to Miller, biological literacy exists along a continuum and varies by education and other types of literacy, such as scientific literacy. Literacy in biology includes recognizing and understanding key terms and concepts and being able to apply them as they relate to the human experience. The ability to examine issues such as genetic mutations and genetically based medicines is important to the discussion of biological literacy (Uno & Bybee, 1994). With respect to cancer, women with low health literacy and/or general literacy may not understand concepts such as triple-negative breast cancer or genetic mutations (e.g., BRCA1 and BRCA2).

Studies estimate that only 16% of adult Americans are biologically literate (Miller, 2007). Health information can overwhelm even persons with advanced literacy skills. Medical science progresses rapidly and what people may have learned about health or biology during their school years becomes outdated or is incomplete. Rapid changes in biological and medical knowledge require adults to have the ability to engage, comprehend, and apply complex information over the lifespan. Without biological literacy, citizens are ill prepared to understand some medical developments and their implications for disease prevention and treatment, from vaccine development and improvement to genomic technologies. Box 1.1 lists health literacy tips for navigators post-COVID.

Health Communication for Colorectal Cancer Screening and Treatment of Low-Income and Racial and Ethnic Communities

Both African Americans and Whites have been shown to have inadequate knowledge of colorectal cancer (CRC) and to be poorly informed about CRC screening and its benefits (Brittain et al., 2016; Greiner et al., 2005), with little information about CRC screening from doctors or the mass media (Beeker et al., 2000). Further, negative attitudes toward screening procedures (Beeker et al., 2000) may perhaps be influenced by fear, which is also a major barrier to screening for African Americans, along with mistrust and fatalism (Beeker et al., 2000; Brittain et al., 2016; Greiner et al., 2005). CRC screening disparities have also been shown between males and females (Green & Kelly, 2004; Yager

Box 1.1 Health Literacy Tips for Navigators Post-COVID

Communications and Instructions

- Think about your patient and her unique COVID-19 risk factors, in addition to her screening and/or cancer treatment needs.
- Assist patients in identifying adequate sources of personal protective equipment to allay fears of returning for screening or treatment.
- Suggest that the woman practice proper mask wearing and removal, as well as social distancing, to increase her sense of efficacy before attending scheduled screening or treatments.
  - Use pictures to help with instructions on proper handwashing technique and mask wearing.
  - Use a medically trained interpreter or translator if a language barrier exists.
  - Identify translations of COVID-19 information, in addition to cancer health and survivor information.
  - Keep it simple. Although the number of messages depends on the needs of the client, attempt to use no more than four main messages:
    - You can safely return for screening and/or care.
    - Discuss the screenings or visits required with your provider.
    - If you have COVID-19 risk factors, request the first appointment of the day to avoid exposures.
    - Focus on healthy behaviors to reduce your risks of cancer and COVID-19.
- Give the woman specific recommendations—for example, "Now is the time to quit smoking to reduce your risk of cancer and COVID-19."
- Clearly state the actions you want the woman to take—for example, return for screening or care.
- Summarize what the client needs to do. Consider using a handout to help her understand screening preparation.
- Leave written instructions. Make sure she knows where the instructions are.
- Check for understanding.
  - Ask the client to repeat the information in her own words.
  - Ask questions using words like "what" or "how"—for example, "What will you do prior to leaving for your screening appointment?"

Written Materials
- Handouts and other printed materials should look easy to read.
- Use at least 12-point font.
- Use headings and bullets to break up text.
- Use cues (arrows, captions) to point out important information.
- Leave plenty of white space around the margins and between sections.

et al., 2014) as well as between urban and non-urban African Americans (Beyer et al., 2011; Cole et al., 2013).

Healthcare delivery disparities have also been shown to influence CRC screening (Preston et al., 2018; Uradamo & Borum, 2011). Many potential barriers to CRC screening exist for the patient and the physician (Dyer et al., 2019; Walsh & Terdiman, 2003). A healthcare provider's recommendation to undergo screening has been shown to be one of the strongest predictors of completing a CRC screening test (Katz et al., 2004). For example, African American participants who rated their patient–provider communication as good were more likely to have completed CRC screening tests than those reporting poor communication (Katz et al., 2004). Among participants reporting good communication, knowledge about CRC was also associated with test completion (Katz et al., 2004). Much of the literature suggests a strong need for increasing knowledge and awareness, including the importance of screening (Green & Kelly, 2004; Nagelhout et al., 2017), by encouraging clinical doctors and healthcare professionals to educate their patients (Agrawal et al., 2005; Green & Kelly, 2004). With regard to targeting educational efforts to African American communities, culturally sensitive health education is needed (Agrawal et al., 2005; Holt et al., 2012) that explains the value of and specific methods used for CRC screening (Thompson Sanders et al., 2010), especially for older African American men and women (Green & Kelly, 2004).

As a part of an effort to understand the role of culture in cancer communication, CRC communication materials were developed for African American women (Thompson Sanders et al., 2010; Figure 1.1). Three full-color publications, 12 pages

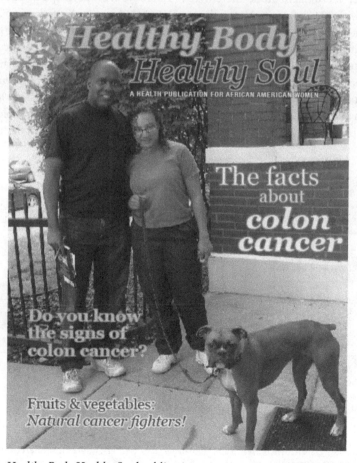

Figure 1.1 *Healthy Body Healthy Soul* publication.

each, were developed. Their content focused on reducing CRC. The publications were sequenced in the following order: (1) beliefs about CRC and screening; (2) dietary behaviors to reduce CRC risk; and (3) CRC screening recommendations (Kreuter et al., 2003; Thompson Sanders et al., 2014a). To understand the role that culture may play in successful CRC awareness and education, two types of magazines were developed: one that used peripheral elements and evidence targeted to African American women and one that incorporated the elements of the first magazine plus references to cultural attitudes and concerns related to cancer (Kreuter et al., 2003; Thompson Sanders et al., 2010). Specifically, evidential screening messages emphasized comparative statistics related to incidence, mortality, and screening rates in the African American community. Sociocultural messages focused on collectivism and ethnic identity through screening appeals that suggested family and community benefit and addressed mistrust and the desire for privacy by emphasizing how these undermined the health of the African American community. Sociocultural peripherals used localized photos and those that depicted church, family, and community scenes.

The study evaluating these materials serves as an example of using a health communication planning process (Figure 1.2). The CRC communication materials were developed as a part of a two-arm randomized controlled trial. The study participants were African Americans between the ages of 45 and 75 years, born in the United States, who lived in the targeted recruitment areas. There were 771 (410 women) participants in the study at baseline, with 702 (388 women), at follow-up 1, 641 (366 women) at follow-up 2, and 600 (348 women) at follow-up 3. Participants were randomly assigned to one of the two publications. The first assessment of the publication was given to participants after completing the baseline survey, with an assessment at 2 weeks; publications were mailed at 10 weeks and 20 weeks, with follow-up telephone calls at 12 and 22 weeks after enrollment.

Participants were recruited from census tracts that were at least 70% African American and had at least 50 houses ($N = 500$). Only one person per household was permitted to participate. Each block was visited three times, varied by time of day and day of

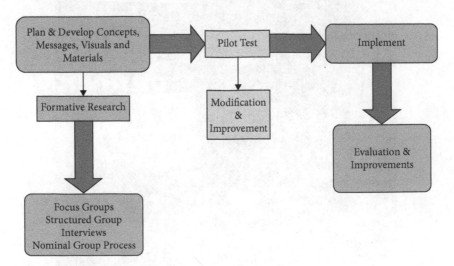

Figure 1.2 Health communication planning process.

Adapted from U.S. Department of Health and Human Services, National Cancer Institute. (2004). *Making health communication programs work*, p. 11.

the week. The individuals recruited were screened for literacy. Individuals who agreed to participate reviewed and signed an informed consent form and received a demographic informational sheet and a baseline survey to complete. Immediately after completion of the baseline survey, research assistants hand-delivered the first CRC publication. Participants were instructed to read the publication prior to the telephone follow-up call.

Interestingly, there were no effects of cultural appropriateness strategy, but there were interactions and findings worth considering when communicating about CRC. The cultural attitudes that proved most important to intervention response were mistrust of the healthcare system and ethnic identity status. If women reported low religiosity, their affective response to the publication was more positive to the peripheral and evidentially focused publication. More religious African American women reported more positive affect toward publications that included sociocultural material. Interestingly, a family history of cancer also interacted with magazine type. Women with no family history of cancer reported less negative affect related to cancer screening in response to the sociocultural publication, while those with a family history of cancer reported less negative affect in response to the peripheral/evidential publication and greater negative affect in response to the sociocultural publication. Sociocultural appeals are personal and relate strongly to group and family protection against cancer, which may be stressful in cases where a family member already has a diagnosis.

Women who reported less mistrust of the healthcare system, adjusting for a sense that there was nothing that could be done about cancer, showed an increase in engagement with the material while reading the sociocultural publication, but the women reading the peripheral/evidential publication did not show an increase in engagement after reading the publication. Among women reporting high mistrust of the healthcare system, the peripheral/evidential publication increased engagement while reading the publication as compared to the sociocultural publication, which showed a reduction in engagement while reading the publication.

Although subtle and dependent upon the individual cultural attitudes and beliefs of members of the target audience, there are differences in affective and cognitive processing responses to peripheral/evidential and sociocultural cancer publications. This intervention failed to demonstrate that the differences observed resulted in changes in intent to obtain CRC screening or screening status. The data do suggest several benefits of sociocultural strategies over peripheral/evidential publications. Sociocultural publications produced a sense of content relevance across ethnic identity statuses; this was not true of peripheral/evidential publications. For this reason, sociocultural publications may have greater utility when ethnic identity status is known to be highly variable in a community. In addition, the sociocultural publications demonstrated some ability to generate positive affective reactions to screening messages among individuals whose racial identity attitudes would suggest the opposite response and be capable of appealing to those for whom mistrust of the healthcare system is an issue without offending those for whom racial identity is not a major issue. Finally, previous studies of the role of culture in cancer communication demonstrated its importance in communications to women (Kreuter et al., 2003). Sociocultural publications may have more appeal in showing the relevance of screening among first-degree relatives and in conveying the ability to care for a family member with cancer. For this reason and because of the strengths of sociocultural publications we have noted, they may be the preferred targeted cancer communication strategy, unless time and/or cost make them prohibitive (Thompson Sanders et al., 2010).

Additional research confirms the relevance of culture in the development of cancer communication and educational materials. The associations among empowerment, collectivism, and privacy items and cancer attitudes and beliefs were strong in a large national sample of African Americans, providing further support for the use of these constructs in cancer and health education activities (Thompson Sanders et al., 2014a). Previous studies have linked collectivism and privacy to cancer attitudes through qualitative analyses (Deshpande et al., 2009). A study by Thompson et al. provided empirical support for the relationship between these constructs and cancer attitudes. The privacy construct appears to have broad associations with cancer attitudes (screening benefits, cancer worry, and perceived cancer risk) that suggest a communication style that may affect African Americans' willingness to discuss feelings and concerns about CRC screening recommendations and information (Thompson Sanders et al., 2014a). Privacy concerns and relationships to social norms suggest that ideas in the African American community that govern the content and level of self-disclosure are important to assess and address in cancer education and behavior interventions. There are also associations among empowerment and self-efficacy, beliefs about the benefits of screening, and cancer worry that may affect screening completion, as well as among collectivism, social norms, and the benefits of screening (Thompson Sanders et al., 2014a). Health educators may find the use of positive frames of health messages, family and group appeals, and community recommendations for collective action useful in encouraging screening and treatment adherence and persistence. In addition, consideration of privacy may assist in identifying communities where health professional communications training will be most useful due to social norms against disclosure of health information.

A streamlined set of issues and concerns that may be relevant for healthcare providers, including nurse navigators, and community health workers supporting patients, and when developing CRC health communication and interventions strategies, were identified using a large, national survey of African Americans' attitudes about cancer and CRC screening (Thompson Sanders et al., 2014b). The issues identified were consistent with factors previously identified in the screening adherence literature—the health practitioner's recommendation to screen, having a risk factor for CRC, and a usual source of care—and are predicted using the Health Belief Model. Knowledge and health practitioner recommendations serve as cues to action for women, risk factors increase the sense of susceptibility to the disease, and a usual source of care can be seen as reducing a barrier to screen. To further verify the relevance of these factors, logistic regressions were completed. Four items classified adherence to CRC screening (53.4% of nonadherent and 83.6% of adherent participants): physician or healthcare provider colonoscopy recommendation, receipt of prevention services at the place healthcare is usually sought, and a history of colitis or polyps (Cox & Snell $R^2 = .14$, Nagelkerke $R^2 = .19$) (Thompson Sanders et al., 2014b). The items that were more strongly associated with nonadherence suggest that nonadherent African American participants without risk factors may not have a perceived sufficient reason to act. The items identified were focused on awareness of a family history of disease and the actual presence of polyps or colitis. These items are in contrast to the focus on physician recommendation and personal disease risk factors noted among those participants who were adherent. It is plausible that the best cancer messages for these individuals highlight the fact that cancer may occur in the absence of family history. The importance of a usual source of care and the receipt of preventive services through that source of care highlight the importance of access concerns that providers, navigators, and community health workers should always be prepared to address (Thompson Sanders et al., 2014b).

In summary, the data suggest that it is important that healthcare providers give a clear recommendation to screen regardless of the method ultimately selected. Healthcare providers, navigators, and community health workers should consider advising African American patients or community members that family history and absence of symptoms do not eliminate the value of screening. In addition, research findings suggest the importance of cultivating the use of a range of preventive health services prior to the age for the initiation of breast cancer, cervical cancer, and CRC screening, as well as human papillomavirus (HPV) vaccination, as these data suggest that individuals who have been adherent to other medical recommendations are more likely to respond to cancer prevention recommendations (Thompson Sanders et al., 2014b).

With respect to promoting HPV vaccination, there were few significant differences among parents who had and who had not vaccinated their daughters (Thompson Sanders et al., 2011). Consistent with prior research, vaccination status was associated with physician recommendation regardless of education. Among those receiving a pediatrician's recommendation for HPV vaccination, approximately 50% of the parents had their daughters vaccinated. Similar to Scarinci et al. (2007), African American parents who had not vaccinated their daughters expressed concerns about vaccine safety, including fears of side effects. Consistent with previous findings, among parents who had not vaccinated their daughters, mistrust of the healthcare system was associated with lack of intent to vaccinate (Dempsey et al., 2006; Micco et al., 2004; Scarinci et al., 2007).

Data suggest that healthcare providers, particularly nurse navigators, and/or community health workers be trained and/or encouraged to consider the recommendations in Box 1.2 (Caito et al., 2014).

Conclusion

Supporting women's autonomy involves communicating in a way that uplifts the patient's sense of efficacy and motivates the woman to take control of her health (Glanz et al., 2008). Much of the support includes exploring women's ambivalence about taking action, providing options, and respectfully allowing them time to consider choices. Good communication between the healthcare provider and the patient can empower women to be more active in improving and managing their health. The provider's goal should be to assist and encourage the woman to have a voice in her own health decisions. This will then help increase self-efficacy so that the woman will being able to manage her own health, giving her a sense of control and confidence when solving problems (be they social, medical, financial, emotional, etc.) and allowing her the volition to follow through with provider recommendations. More empowered women feel more control over their disease, which has been linked to emotional well-being and coping during treatment (Nikbakht Nasrabadi et al., 2015).

For many of us, the way we practice as healthcare providers today has changed from a decade ago and will likely change significantly over the next decade or so. These changes suggest that we need to be better at communicating with our patients. Communication is also how patients find a doctor, describe their symptoms, understand the diagnosis we offer them, share information, learn about treatment plans, and make decisions about

---

Box 1.2 Communication Tips

General Preparation and Communication

1. Understand your healthcare system's history and relationships with racial/ethnic and low-income communities, particularly situations and experiences that may stimulate or inform mistrust.
2. Attempt to understand the patient's cancer-related beliefs and attitudes that are relevant to screening, treatment decision-making, and adherence.
3. Demonstrate respect by listening, acknowledging the woman's fears and concerns, and responding to the questions she poses without judgment.
4. Discuss family, personal, and financial stress, and ways to cope collaboratively.
5. Consider how to be supportive of the use of spirituality/religion as a coping strategy or source of support when dealing with fears or anxieties related to screening, diagnosis, or health concerns.
6. Collaborate to find food preparation methods and foods, exercise routines, and smoking cessation programs that support health and are affordable, accessible, community focused, and/or culturally sensitive.

Cancer-Specific Communication and Support

1. Use lay or community terms paired with cancer terminology to increase familiarity and comfort with the medical terminology.
2. Make or seek explicit cancer screening and HPV vaccination recommendations (from physicians or other healthcare providers), particularly when appropriate due to age or family history.
3. Use a positive frame: "These tests allow us to see if your breasts/colon is healthy" versus "These tests allow us to screen for cancer."
4. Educate patients and carefully explain tests, test preparation, costs, and pros and cons. Identify and share resources to make screening affordable or accessible.
5. Use layman's terms to explain that if cancer is found, individuals can be treated immediately to increase their chances of survival.
6. Discuss what happens after a positive screening, such as treatment options, assistance obtaining needed services, specific actions that will be provided, and support that can be offered.
7. Be prepared to discuss what is known about the efficacy of treatments, screening, medication, and so forth. Use nontechnical language.

Caito et al., 2014; Kreuter et al., 2003; Thompson et al., 2010; Thompson Sanders et al., 2011.

---

their health. Thus, making sure that we communicate effectively is critical, sometimes even a matter of life or death.

References

Agrawal, S., Bhupinderjit, A., Bhutani, M. S., Boardman, L., Nguyen, C., Romero, Y., Srinvasan, R., & Figueroa-Moseley, C. (2005). Colorectal cancer in African Americans. *American Journal of Gastroenterology, 100,* 515–523. 10.1111/j.1572 0241.2005.41829.x

Beeker, C., Kraft, J. M., Southwell, B. G., & Jorgensen, C. M. (2000). Colorectal cancer screening in older men and women: Qualitative research findings and implications for intervention. *Journal of Community Health, 25*, 263–278.

Benjamin, R. M. (2010). Improving health by improving health literacy. *Public Health Reports (Washington, D.C.: 1974), 125*(6), 784–785. doi:10.1177/003335491012500602

Betancourt, J. R., & Tan-McGrory, A. (2014). Creating a safe, high-quality healthcare system for all: Meeting the needs of limited English proficient populations; Comment on "Patient safety and healthcare quality: The case for language access." *International Journal of Health Policy and Management, 2*(2), 91–94. doi:10.15171/ijhpm.2014.21

Beyer, K. M. M., Comstock, S., Seagren, R., & Rushton, G. (2011). Explaining place-based colorectal cancer health disparities: Evidence from a rural context. *Social Science & Medicine, 72*(3), 373–382.

Brittain, K., Christy, S. M., & Rawl, S. M. (2016). African American patients' intent to screen for colorectal cancer: Do cultural factors, health literacy, knowledge, age, and gender matter? *Journal of Health Care for the Poor and Underserved, 27*(1), 51–67.

Cabana, M. D., & Jee, S. H. (2004). Does continuity of care improve patient outcomes? *Journal of Family Practice, 53*(12), 974–980.

Caito, N., Hood, S., & Thompson Sanders, V. L. (2014). Discussing cancer: Communication with African Americans. *Social Work in Health Care, 53*, 519–531.

Centers for Disease Control and Prevention. (2016). What is health literacy? https://www.cdc.gov/healthliteracy/learn/index.html

Cole, A. M., Jackson, J. E., & Doescher, M. (2013). Colorectal cancer screening disparities for rural minorities in the United States. *Journal of Primary Care & Community Health, 4*(2), 106–111.

Committee on Improving the Quality of Cancer Care: Addressing the Challenges of an Aging Population; Board on Health Care Services; Institute of Medicine. (2013). Patient-centered communication and shared decision making. In L. Levit, E. Balogh, S. Nass, & P. A. Glanz (Eds.), *Delivering high-quality cancer care: Charting a new course for a system in crisis* (pp. 91–152)National Academies Press.

Dempsey, A. F., Zimet, G. D., Davis, R. L., & Koutsky, L. (2006). Factors that are associated with parental acceptance of human papillomavirus vaccines: A randomized intervention study of written information about HPV. *Pediatrics, 117*(5), 1486–1493.

Deshpande, A. D., Thompson Sanders, V. L., Vaughn, K. P., & Kreuter, M. W. (2009). Use of socio-cultural constructs in cancer research among African Americans: A review. *Cancer Control, 16*(3), 256–265.

Dyer, K. E., Shires, D. A., Flocke, S. A., Hawley, S. T., Jones, R. M., Resnicow, K., Shin, Y., & Lafata, J. E. (2019). Patient-reported needs following a referral for colorectal cancer screening. *American Journal of Preventive Medicine, 56*(2), 271–280.

Fuertes, J. N., Mislowack, A., Bennett, J., Paul, L., Gilbert, T. C., Fontan, G., & Boylan, L. S. (2007). The physician–patient working alliance. *Patient Education and Counseling, 66*, 29–36.

Glanz, K., Rimer, B. K., & Viswanath, K. (Eds.). (2008). *Health behavior and health education: Theory, research, and practice* (4th ed.). Jossey-Bass.

Gordon, H. S., Street, R. L., Sharf, B. F., & Souchek, J. (2006). Racial differences in doctors' information-giving and patient participation. *Cancer, 107*(6), 1313–1320. doi:10.1002/cncr.22122

Green, P. M., & Kelly, B. A. (2004). Colorectal cancer knowledge, perceptions, and behaviors in African Americans. *Cancer Nursing, 27*, 206–215. doi:10.1097/00002820-200405000 00004

Greiner, K. A., Born, W., Nollen, N., & Ahluwalia, J. S. (2005). Knowledge and perceptions of colorectal cancer screening among urban African Americans. *Journal of General Internal Medicine, 20*(11), 977–983. doi:10.1111/j.1525-1497.2005.00165.x

Healthy People 2030. (2021). U.S. Department of Health and Human Services, Office of Disease Prevention and Health Promotion. https://health.gov/healthypeople/objectives-and-data/social-determinants-health

Holt, C. L., Scarinci, I. C., Debnam, K., McDavid, C., Litaker, M., McNeal, S. F., Southward, V., Lee, C., Eloubeidi, M., Crowther, M., Bolland, J., & Martin, M. Y. (2012). Spiritually based intervention to increase colorectal cancer awareness among African Americans: Intermediate outcomes from a randomized trial. *Journal of Health Communication, 17*(9), 1028–1049.

Jongen, C., McCalman, J., & Bainbridge, R. (2018). Health workforce cultural competency interventions: A systematic scoping review. *BMC Health Services Research, 18*(1), 232. doi:10.1186/s12913-018-3001-5

Ka'opua, L. S., Park, S. H., Ward, M. E., & Braun, K. L. (2011). Testing the feasibility of a culturally tailored breast cancer screening intervention with Native Hawaiian women in rural churches. *Health & Social Work, 36*(1), 55–65. doi:10.1093/hsw/36.1.55

Katz, M. L., James, A. S., & Pignone, M. P. (2004). Colorectal cancer screening among African American church members: A qualitative and quantitative study of patient-provider communication. *BMC Public Health, 4*, 62.

Kreps, G. L. (2006). Communication and racial inequities in health care. *American Behavioral Scientist, 49*(6), 760–774. doi:10.1177/0002764205283800

Kreuter, M., Lukwago, S., Bucholtz, D., Clark, E., & Thompson Sanders, V. (2003). Achieving cultural appropriateness in health promotion programs: Targeted and tailored approaches. *Health Education & Behavior, 30*, 133–146.

Lee, H. Y., Rhee, T. G., Kim, N. K., & Ahluwalia, J. S. (2015). Health literacy as a social determinant of health in Asian American immigrants: Findings from a population-based survey in California. *Journal of General Internal Medicine, 30*(8), 1118–1124.

Limited English Proficiency. (2021). *Commonly asked questions.* https://lep.gov/commonly-asked-questions

Micco, E., Gurmankin, A., & Armstrong, K. (2004). Differential willingness to undergo smallpox vaccination among African American and White individuals. *Journal of General Internal Medicine, 19*(5 pt 1), 451–455.

Miller, J. (2007). *Assessing the public's comprehension of biomedical science.* Paper presented at the HINTS Data Users Conference, Pasadena, CA, May 4–5.

Nagelhout, E., Comarell, K., Samadder, N. J., & Wu, Y. P. (2017). Barriers to colorectal cancer screening in a racially diverse population served by a safety-net clinic. *Journal of Community Health, 42*(4), 791–796.

National Center for Education Statistics. (2006). *The health literacy of America's adults: Results from the 2003 National Assessment of Adult Literacy.* U.S. Department of Education.

Nikbakht Nasrabadi, A., Sabzevari, S., & Negahban Bonabi, T. (2015). Women empowerment through health information seeking: A qualitative study. *International Journal of Community-Based Nursing and Midwifery, 3*(2), 105–115.

Ohio Mental Health and Addiction Services. (2019). *Cultural competence in mental health and addiction recovery.* Ohio eBased Academy.

O'Toole, J. K., Alvarado-Little, W., & Ledford, C. J. W. (2019). Communication with diverse patients: Addressing culture and language. *Pediatric Clinics of North America, 66*(4), 791–804.

Preston, M. A., Glover-Collins, K., Ross, L., Porter, A., Bursac, Z., Woods, D., Burton, J., Crowell, K., Laryea, J., & Henry-Tillman, R. (2018). Colorectal cancer screening in rural and poor-resourced communities. *American Journal of Surgery, 216*(2), 245–250.

Scarinci, I. C., Garces-Palacio, I. C., & Partridge, E. E. (2007). An examination of acceptability of HPV vaccination among African American women and Latina immigrants. *Journal of Women's Health, 16*(8), 1224–1233.

Thompson Sanders, V. L., Arnold, L., & Notaro, S. (2011). African American parents' attitudes toward HPV vaccination. *Ethnicity & Disease, 21*(3), 335–341.

Thompson Sanders, V. L., Harris, J., Clark, E. M., Purnell, J., & Deshpande, A. D. (2014a). Broadening the examination of socio-cultural constructs relevant to African American colorectal cancer screening. *Psychology, Health & Medicine, 20*(1), 47–58. doi10.1080/13548506.2014.894639

Thompson Sanders, V. L., Kalesan, B., Wells, A., Williams, S-L., & Caito, N. (2010). Comparing the use of evidence and culture in targeted colorectal cancer communication for African Americans. *Patient Education and Counseling, 81*(S1), S22–S33. doi:10.1016/j.pec.2010.07.019

Thompson Sanders, V., Lander, S., Xu, S., & Shyu, C. (2014b). Identifying key variables in African American adherence to colorectal cancer screening: The application of data mining. *BMC: Public Health, 14*, 1173. doi:10.1186/1471-2458-14-1173

Uno, G. E., & Bybee, R. W. (1994). Understanding the dimensions of biological literacy. *Bioscience, 44*(8), 553–557.

Uradamo, L., Mener, A., & Borum, M. (2011). Insurance coverage for screening colonoscopy at age 45 for African Americans: Low adherence to guidelines in states with large African American populations. Paper presented at Digestive Diseases Week.

Vermeir, P., Vandijck, D., Degroote, S., Peleman, R., Verhaeghe, R., Mortier, E., & Vogelaers, D. (2015). Communication in healthcare: A narrative review of the literature and practical recommendations. *International Journal of Clinical Practice, 69*(11), 1257–1267. doi:10.1111/ijcp.12686

Walsh, J. M., & Terdiman, J. P. (2003). Colorectal cancer screening: Scientific review. *Journal of the American Medical Association, 289*, 1288–1296. doi:10.1001/jama.289.10.1288

Wells, A., Sanders Thompson, V. L., Camp Yeakey, C., & Notaro, S. (2019). *Poverty and place: Cancer prevention among low-income women of color.* Lexington Books.

Wilson, C. C. (2013). Patient safety and healthcare quality: The case for language access. *International Journal of Health Policy and Management, 1*(4), 251–253. doi:10.15171/ijhpm.2013.53

Wolf, M. S., Davis, T. C., & Parker, R. M. (2007). Editorial: The emerging field of health literacy research. *American Journal of Health Behavior, 31*(Supplement 1), S3–S5.

Yager, S. S., Chen, L., & Cheung, W. Y. (2014). Sex-based disparities in colorectal cancer screening. *American Journal of Clinical Oncology, 37*(6), 555–560.

Module 1.2: Recognizing and Assessing Adherence Barriers and Stressors

This module discusses how to recognize and assess barriers and stressors, including the full range of factors that can get in the way of preventive screening and cancer care. We cover challenges facing women that often make it difficult to follow up with care, such as financial strain, insurance concerns, housing problems, physical and mental health issues, legal problems, caregiving demands, underemployment or unemployment, employment commitments, and problems accessing healthcare systems. Also described are organizational barriers, such as mistreatment on the part of healthcare providers and discrimination. These real-world barriers and stressors become apparent in two sample cases. "If/then" examples will provide possible responses for the provider.

Addressing barriers and stressors is essential to effective implementation of the expanded CCM. Given that the Heath Disparities Collaboratives were developed to eliminate health disparities, expanded CCM must take into account the barriers that contribute to disparities in order to find solutions for them and to improve outcomes. This module will vividly illustrate the characteristics of low-income women of color. We begin our discussion of general screening adherence barriers, focusing on common barriers and facilitators among African American women. As providers ourselves, we have listened to the challenges, frustrations, and practical demands of frontline providers trying to address general medical adherence barriers:

I am a nurse case manager working in a multidisciplinary team in an infectious disease clinic. I have a 26-year-old female who was diagnosed with HIV five years ago. She reports an interest in her health when she is in need of medication, but yet she does not take it as prescribed. She has had a decrease in her CD4 [count and] immune system and has had an increase in her viral load. She has not seen the doctor consistently. She has also had an increase in STDs over the last year. We have repeatedly discussed her meds; she reports taking them, then later states she has missed multiple [doses]. She states her partner does not believe in medication and she has to hide her meds from her partner when she takes them.

I am a medical social worker working on an interdisciplinary team in an outpatient clinic that serves people who are low income and uninsured or underinsured. I have a 34-year-old female patient with uncontrolled diabetes, diabetic retinopathy, diabetic neuropathy, hyperlipidemia, and hypertension. She has been noncompliant with medications, diet, and checking blood sugars. The dietitian was consulted when [the] patient was first diagnosed in her late teens. The clinical pharmacist has been working closely with this patient for almost three years, I have been working with her for two years, and the community health nurse has been making home visits for the past year, but the patient continues to be noncompliant. We have talked at length about the emotional issues that may be playing a role in her noncompliance, to no avail. She provides no insights or possible future consequences such as amputations and dialysis to motivate her to change her lifestyle and be compliant with her medications.

I am a medical case manager that works on an interdisciplinary team within a clinic setting. I carry a general and a specialty caseload; my specialty caseload is for clients who need nursing home–level care. I have a 41-year-old female client who is part of my specialty caseload. She lives independently in an apartment with her adult children and receives five hours/day in home health care. The client's health was not good and the apartment complex gave her a few months to get back on her feet. Her health has not improved and she recently had a seizure and hit her head. The apartment complex has given her the option of moving into supportive housing to improve her health, while still allowing her children to maintain the apartment. If the client chooses not to go into supportive housing, her housing with the apartment complex will be terminated.

The client reports that she does not want to move into supportive housing temporarily because she does not want to leave her children.

Often women sacrifice adherence in order to take care of their families. Adherence (the extent to which women follow screening and treatment recommendations) barriers include individual/sociocultural factors, tensions in the patient–provider relationship, and organizational/structural complications that make systems difficult to navigate. These barriers represent obstacles for women's adherence to diagnostic follow-up, such as "catch-up" human papillomavirus (HPV) vaccination completion, Papanicolaou (Pap) screening for cervical cancer, and post-screening/diagnostic follow-up recommendations after an abnormal Pap test (Bernard et al., 2012; Horner et al., 2011; Misra-Herbert et al., 2017; Tejeda et al., 2013). Nonadherence following an abnormal screen and/or cancer diagnosis is often the result of psychological, sociocultural, and environmental "place" barriers. If the woman's perception of the process is more painful than what you "think" you have (e.g., cancer), then you tend to delay. It has been shown that women who have never been screened or are less knowledgeable about screening guidelines have inaccurate beliefs, have competing needs, lack social support, have poor access to care, and are less likely to use healthcare services or have a recommendation from a healthcare provider (Talley et al., 2017). To improve follow-up rates, providers must be aware of these barriers, especially given that many of these barriers are at the system level and providers are often responsible for performing the initial screening. What we still need are better interventions to help understand and address the barriers and facilitators contributing to adherence among at-risk low-income women of color.

Adherence Barriers and Facilitators: Breast Cancer Treatment Among African American Women

Equally important to the discussion of diagnostic delay in treatment is the problem of failing to follow up on treatment recommendations *after* an abnormal breast examination and diagnosis occurs. African American women are reportedly less likely than other groups of women to use healthcare services despite an equal or greater need (Baker & Jemmott, 2014; Copeland et al., 2003). African American breast cancer survivors have been shown to be the least likely to receive adjuvant therapies, including radiation and chemotherapy (Paladino et al., 2019), as compared to Asians and Latinas (Ashing-Giwa et al., 2004). Numerous studies have examined population-based cancer screening programs to detect cancer early, but far fewer have examined the issue of adherence with follow-up examinations subsequent to suggestive findings (Richardson & Sanchez, 1998). Discussion of follow-up adherence to cancer treatment requires the consideration of timeliness of accessing treatment because cancer stage is the most important determinant of survival (Caplan & Helzlsouer, 1992-93; Richardson & Sanchez, 1998; Selove et al., 2016). The timeliness of this type of follow-up treatment is often influenced by the individual's knowledge of the importance of the treatment; her own or her family's or friends' experience with a cancer diagnosis and treatment; access to medical care and treatment; and numerous other psychological, sociodemographic, and cultural factors (Marouf, 2020; Richardson & Sanchez, 1998). Another common and non–patient-related problem is system delay (Caplan & Helzlsouer, 1992-93; Nonzee et al., 2015). Thus, it is essential to treatment adherence and follow-up for breast cancer among

African American women for providers to understand the structural barriers and corresponding psychosocial strategies at the individual, cultural, and healthcare system levels (Bradley, 2005; Caplan & Helzlsouer, 1992-93; Whyte, 2000).

Cultural values and perceptions can also influence adherence to treatment, with perceived severity and perceived barriers found to be significantly related to clinical breast examination and mammography (Beckjord & Klassen, 2008; McDonald et al., 1999; Wang et al., 2009). For example, in a sample of African American women with breast cancer, more traditional cultural values were associated with worse screening histories and lower intentions for future breast cancer screening (Beckjord & Klassen, 2008). And in another study, a sample of African American women residing in public housing did not perceive themselves or a particular racial or economic group to be more susceptible to breast cancer (McDonald et al., 1999). Moreover, the women in the sample did not perceive breast cancer as a fatal disease and also denied the relevance of commonly cited barriers to breast cancer screening (McDonald et al., 1999). An understanding of cultural factors is important in increasing screening and treatment adherence and thus reducing breast cancer disparities for African American women (Beckjord & Klassen, 2008; Talley et al., 2017).

African American women often describe spiritual and support coping mechanisms as the most important sociocultural *facilitators* to breast cancer treatment adherence at various stages along the cancer care continuum (Ashing-Giwa, 1999; Gibson & Hendricks, 2006; Henderson et al., 2003; Schulz, 2008). As such, African American women's decisions about mammography screening and treatment are associated with prayer and relying on religious beliefs and social supports (including family members, spouses, church, and support groups) (Fowler, 2006a; Sage et al., 2020).

Spirituality is associated with health and well-being and plays an important role in mammography utilization and cancer treatment decisions (Gullate, 2006; Holt et al., 2003b; Sage et al., 2020). The mechanism through which this occurs involves the pathway from spiritual perspective through hope and psychological well-being (Richardson Gibson & Parker, 2003). Breast cancer survivors, particularly women of color, often voice that their spiritual beliefs and practices are central to their coping (Ashing-Giwa et al., 2004; Bourjolly, 1998; Henderson et al., 2003; Lynn et al., 2014). Latino women have also reported more religious coping than non-Latino Whites (Culver et al., 2002). It is believed that spiritually based approaches may be one way to make cancer communication more culturally appropriate for African American women, as it is an important component in their lives (Holt et al., 2003a, 2003b; Sheppard et al., 2018). For example, African American women who were eligible for tamoxifen prophylaxis (an estrogen-blocking treatment for patients with increased risk of breast cancer) because of their breast cancer risk described faith as important to preventing and reducing their risk of breast cancer (Paterniti et al., 2005). Fatalism, related to the concept of spirituality, has been contributed to the delay in screening among African American women with breast cancer, leading to advanced-stage cancer diagnosis (Gullatte et al., 2010; Mitchell et al., 2002). African American women often believe that medical treatment is unnecessary because only God (who works through doctors) can cure breast cancer (labeled "religious intervention in place of treatment") (Mitchell et al., 2002). Thus, understanding that spiritual belief systems can be used as culturally appropriate forms of intervention has important implications for cancer communication interventions that involve spirituality (Holt et al., 2003b; Sage et al., 2020).

Social relationships and networks and strong interdependence within the extended family system are primary cancer coping resources in African American and Latino communities (Flannery et al., 2019; Meyerowitz et al., 2000; Wilmoth & Sanders, 2001). Social support also serves as a vital facilitator to treatment decision-making and coping throughout the breast cancer continuum. African American women's decisions about mammography screening are associated with valuing the opinions of significant others (Fowler, 2006; Jones, 2015; Pasick & Burke, 2008). Family members also have significant influence over African American women's illness-related self-care activities (Flannery et al., 2019; Warren-Findlow & Prohaska, 2008). With regard to cancer screening behaviors, family networks are associated with both cancer screening recency and the intention to screen for cancer (Klassen & Washington, 2008). As such, social roles and networks have been shown to be positively associated with both emotional support and cancer screening knowledge (Klassen & Washington, 2008; Pullen et al., 2014). Importantly, cancer places new stress on the social system, so patients may require additional support (Meyerowitz et al., 2000). This is especially important as African American breast cancer survivors reported difficulty talking about the disease on the one hand and a lack of adequate emotional and functional support on the other (Ashing-Giwa, 1999; Ashing-Giwa et al., 2004).

African American women and White women with breast cancer tend to seek social support as a way of coping with their breast cancer, but they may differ in their sources of support (Bourjolly & Hirschman, 2001; Paladino et al., 2019). In particular, African Americans rely more frequently on informal sources of healthcare advice such as family members and/or social support networks (Copeland et al., 2003). Research on social support suggests that it is not the number of social contacts or that the contacts are necessarily from one's family but rather the quality of the relationship that influences the individual's ability to cope with distress and adhere to treatment. African American breast cancer survivors describe various positive sources of support: *family members*, particularly *spouses*, their *church*, and *support groups* (Copeland et al., 2003; Henderson et al., 2003; Klassen & Washington, 2008; Morgan et al., 2005a, 2005b, 2006; Wallner et al., 2017; Warren-Findlow & Prohaska, 2008; Whyte, 2000; Wilmoth & Sanders, 2001). Given African American sociocultural traditions of spirituality and various informal social support networks, churches should be considered an ideal venue for African American breast cancer survivors, as churches are known to offer a solid support network and are often willing to offer the use of the church for health meetings or support groups (Henderson et al., 2003; Wells et al., 2014; Whyte, 2000; Wilmoth & Sanders, 2001). Thus, it is important to identify the nature of the patient's support rather than its mere presence, based on the context of the patient's life and her sociocultural preferences, because this can be an important factor in mitigating emotional problems in cancer patients and facilitating treatment adherence (Davis et al., 2016; McDaniel et al., 1995; Meichenbaum & Turk, 1987).

Adherence Barriers and Stressors

We acknowledge the distinct stressor characteristics of low-income women of color, which make it difficult to adhere to cancer care preventive guidelines. Often these women are seeking assistance with basic human needs like paying for shelter, utilities, a job, or food. In the face of acute life challenges like these, it is easy to see how cancer screening might not be a woman's highest priority and could create even more stress. Stressors that we see among these women can be categorized into acute life events, chronic socioeconomic strain, trauma, and discrimination.

We present descriptions of women's psychosocial needs, stressors, and barriers in preventive cancer care. We show the full range of stressors and barriers reported by women that might interfere with behaviors like getting a mammogram or Pap test. Such barriers can be categorized into Turner and Avison's (2003) stress exposure list, which comprises recent life events, chronic stressors, lifetime major events, and discrimination stress, and has been tested with minority and low-income groups (Wells et al., 2019).

Recent Life Events

Women in need of mammogram screening or Pap testing found **recent life events**, or things that happened to them or a person close to them in the past 12 months, to be barriers:

- *Finances and insurance*: inability to pay for utilities or having them disconnected, facing foreclosure, being denied Medicare, and becoming recently uninsured
- *Job-related stress*: recent unemployment
- *Housing situations*: severe weather damage to home, relocation to a new home in a new city, recent homelessness, poor living conditions, and general housing stress
- *Physical and mental health issues*: recent hospitalization, recent injury or surgery, diagnosis of disease, general physical health issues, and substance addiction
- *Legal issues*: being under house arrest and carjacking/robbery
- *Caregiving demands*: serving as a caregiver for relatives, letting their own health care needs go unmet.

Chronic Stress

Chronic stress, which is often found in conjunction with recent life events, involves situations that recur in a woman's life. They cause stress and strain on the woman and ultimately are a barrier to receiving proper mammography screening and Pap testing:

- *Financial strain*: inability to obtain assistance with food/utilities or rent/mortgage payment, insufficient money for emergencies, bankruptcy, inability to pay for clothing and infant needs, and lack of health insurance
- *Unemployment/employment commitment*: unemployment and working multiple jobs
- *Housing problems*: landlord issues, unsafe/unsanitary living conditions, homelessness, moving in with family or friends, and strained relationships
- *Problems accessing healthcare systems*: difficulty finding time for appointments, long wait times to see the doctor, lack of transportation, living in a rural area without nearby health providers, and trouble navigating healthcare/social service system
- *Physical health*: dental/vision problems, trying to quit smoking, inability to work due to disability, general fear of doctors, and chronic pain from illness/accident
- *Mental/emotional/addiction issues*: depression; stress; drugs/alcoholism; other mental illness; trying to quit smoking; addiction recovery; fear of doctors, mammograms, and/or mammogram results
- *Legal issues*: lack of legal assistance
- *Caregiver issues*: providing care for ill and/or elderly relatives.

Major Lifetime Events

Major lifetime events, or life trauma, are more serious events that could have happened at any time and had a significant impact on the individual. There are three categories:

- *Illness/disability*: disease diagnosis, poor disability prognosis, and/or an accident resulting in permanent disability
- *Family member's death/loss*: miscarriage, a cancer death in the family, or a sudden death of a relative
- *Other traumatic psychosocial issues*: domestic violence, molestation, shame related to rape, and negative healthcare experiences.

Discrimination Stress

Finally, **discrimination stress** involves biased and/or unfair treatment experienced from other people, such as a previous bad experience with clinic staff or not being treated fairly at a medical facility.

Multiple confounding barriers seemed to contribute to some low-income minority women not being able to continue with cancer screening or treatment. As was identified with most barriers, it is often difficult to extract the sole reason for the woman not continuing with treatment. Stressors and barriers overlap and often influence one another. For example, language-related barriers and perceived discriminatory barriers can often be described as combined experiences, as well as dissatisfaction with screening options and provider issues. This multiplicity of barriers often creates the sense that there were indirect barrier links instead of strong direct links (Rice et al., 2018). This multiplicity of factors suggests that intensive case management may be useful early in cancer treatment to address pressing instrumental issues. Perhaps if these issues are effectively addressed early on (as is often suggested by providers), women will be more likely to present for screening and remain in treatment.

It is just as important to help women navigate the demanding world of cancer treatment. Cancer treatment can cause major disruptions to a woman's daily routine, especially in a large public-sector care system where there are often long waiting periods for appointments. It can have a ripple effect into other life commitments and demands (e.g., making lifestyle changes like exercising more or adhering to a better diet). These multiple stressors become especially important when discussing cancer treatment barriers (Nickell et al., 2019). In women receiving cancer treatment, the aggressiveness of the treatment regimen, its side effects, its impact on their general physical health, and the disruptions it causes to their routine and lifestyle; their level of understanding about the treatment plan; their age and point in the life cycle; their tolerance of uncertainty; their problem-solving capacity; their relationship with the healthcare team; and the availability of social support will collectively influence their ability to manage the rigors of therapy (Lang et al., 2018; Wells & Turney, 2001). Given that cancer treatment barriers can affect both those in active treatment and those who require additional medical appointments with doctors, it is especially important for providers and clinicians to be flexible (Banegas et al, 2018), such as by rescheduling appointments when the patient is not feeling well or misses appointments; arranging late afternoon and weekend appointments to accommodate patients or family members on whom the patient is dependent for transportation to the clinic; and finding a private available room within the busy, often noisy clinic setting (Davey et al., 2016; Ell et al., 2007). Being flexible may facilitate treatment retention.

Relevant to the discussion of stressors and barriers is how a woman's comorbid medical problems can interfere with her treatment follow-through. Comorbid chronic diseases are common in persons with cancer, and the prevalence of comorbidity has important clinical, health service, and research implications (Cofie et al., 2018; Ogle et al.,

2000). Healthcare providers working with nonadherent women and cancer patients need to be prepared to work with other psychosocial issues related to comorbid illnesses. Below are two case studies that reflect the multiple confounding stressors and barriers that can interfere with screening, diagnostic testing, and treatment.

Case 1: Ms. Smith

Ms. Smith is a 58-year-old divorced African American woman with a four-year history of type 2 diabetes (Box 1.3). Records indicate that she has never had a mammogram. She reports fear about the procedure "causing cancer," as both her sister and grandmother died of breast cancer in their mid-40s after receiving a mammogram, chemotherapy, and radiation treatment. Due to her age and family history, doctors have advised her to have a screening, although she does not believe these tests are necessary because she had an older sister and aunt die of breast cancer despite getting a mammogram. Although her mother (age 75) is still alive, her healthy is declining due to some chronic health problems (e.g., diabetes, chronic obstructive pulmonary disease [COPD], hypertension). She reports that she is unfamiliar with her father's medical history. She has one estranged son, whom she has not seen or had any known knowledge about for the past 18-plus years. Although Ms. Smith is very religious and attends a local Baptist church and prayer group regularly, she is a very private person and does not have close friends.

Ms. Smith formerly owned a small business, but following the recession she lost her business and her source of income. For the past 10 years, she has been struggling financially and, without the stable emotional support of friends and family, she fears the onset of additional costs. Although she might be eligible for Medicaid, she has not signed up for health insurance coverage, so she has to go to a Federally Qualified Health Clinic

---

Box 1.3 Case of Ms. Smith

Ms. Smith
Age: 58
Race: African American
Marital status: Divorced

Medical History
Diabetes
Fasting glucose level 168 mg/dL (normal range: 65–109 mg/dL)
A1C value 7.8% (normal: 4–6%)
Breast cancer (sister, grandmother)
COPD (mother)
Hypertension (mother)

Family History
Mother has multiple medical problems.
Grandmother and sister died of breast cancer.

(FQHC) for medical care. She currently works parttime at a local department store, where she assists customers in finding products using iPads and other electronic devices. However, for the past year, she notes increasing difficulty viewing the screen and often quotes incorrect prices to customers as a result of her fluctuating vision. In the past, healthcare providers have attributed her early retinopathy to unstable blood glucose levels. While she has been able to maneuver through these hindrances, she has not been to work for the past month as a result of increasing numbness in her feet and toes, as well as swelling of her ankles, making it exceedingly difficult to walk and further jeopardizing her source of income.

At the recommendation of two female co-workers around the same age, she made an appointment for a physical exam and a mammogram/mammography screening appointment. She was seen for the physical exam, at which time the physician recommended that she start on insulin. She missed the mammogram/mammography screening appointment due to "not feeling well." She has not returned phone messages to reschedule.

What possible multidisciplinary interventions would be important for Ms. Smith (Figure 1.3)?

- Schedule mammogram/mammography screening
- Lifestyle modifications through diet and physical activity to prevent further complications
- Apply for health insurance
- Address barriers to care:
  - Eligibility for home care?
  - Physical therapy/occupational therapy assessment to evaluate for self-care ability
  - Insulin affordability?
  - Insulin adherence?
  - Limited access to healthy diet and physical activity?
  - Limited social support?
  - Eligibility for community resources?

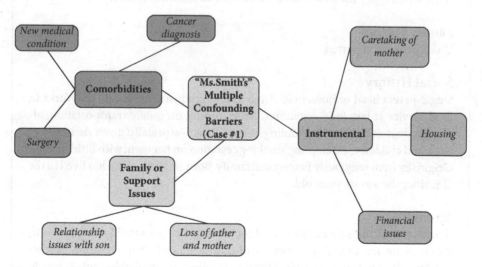

Figure 1.3 Ms. Smith's stressors and barriers.

- Transportation to appointments?
- Depression and/or anxiety?
- Address other comorbidities by referring to specialty providers (e.g., eye care professional, social worker, dentist)
- Provide education and support by telephone.

Case 2: Maria

Maria is a 36-year-old Mexican-born (she reports she immigrated to the United States when she was six years old) mother of three who has received an abnormal Pap screening two months ago (Box 1.4). Her doctor advised her to return to the clinic for a diagnostic

---

Box 1.4 Case of Maria

Maria
Age: 36
Race: Hispanic/Latina
Marital status: Single

Medical History
Abnormal Pap 2 months prior
Overweight
Diabetes mellitus type 2
Regular smoker (0.5 pack/day)

Medications
Review DM type 2 medications and access/medication adherence.

Family History
Unknown or unreported

Social History
Single-parent head of household. High school graduate, some college. Works in food service at fast-food restaurant. Relies mostly on public transportation, although does own a car. Scheduling is a challenge, especially given demands of work and childcare. Attempting smoking cessation on her own, with little success. Originally from religiously Pentecostal family. Born in Mexico, but has lived in the U.S. since she was six years old.

Strengths
Maria's role as the sole caregiver and provider of her household can be a motivating factor for attending to her own healthcare needs. Support from brother and friends sometimes available. Owns a car (albeit an unreliable one). Access to public resources such as nearby park, public transport.

---

test. She has scheduled two appointments but has missed them both. She expressed intent to come in for her test, but has "not been able to." During her pregnancies, Maria accessed low-cost prenatal care at a nearby Planned Parenthood clinic, where she received most of her medical care. She mentioned that she went to these appointments alone or accompanied by her partner at the time, since she did not want her family or friends to find out she was attending a Planned Parenthood clinic; she was worried about "causing tension" with her parents, who she mentions are Pentecostal Christians. This sometimes made it difficult to keep appointments, as she couldn't easily reach out for support from family or friends to help with transportation or, later on, looking after her older children while she went to appointments. Since her last pregnancy five years ago, her access to medical care has been more sporadic.

Maria has comorbid health problems: She is overweight, has type 2 diabetes, and smokes a half-pack of cigarettes per day. She is single, head of household, and lives with her three school-age children in a two-bedroom apartment in a low-income, urban area in a Midwestern city. Maria is a high school graduate, with some college. She works as a server in a 24-hour fast-food restaurant, approximately 10 miles away from home. She maintains this job because "the tips are really good." She uses the metro bus to commute. Although she has a car, it is somewhat unreliable at times; she prefers to use the metro for commuting to work or for important appointments. The local area lacks access to grocery stores and other fresh, healthy food establishments. At times in the past few months, Maria has had to use food pantries in the area or rely on support from her brother and friends when they are able to provide. However, she reports that she feels "ashamed" of having to rely on others, especially when she knows that many of her friends also face financial challenges. On breaks from work, Maria often goes for lunch at various fast-food restaurants. Maria likes to walk at a nearby park when the weather is nice, but she does not get as much exercise during the cold weather months. She sometimes tries to walk around her neighborhood but states that sometimes she doesn't "feel comfortable" doing so.

Maria is a half-pack-a-day smoker. She has been trying to reduce her use, especially due to the cost of cigarettes, but she finds it difficult to resist cravings and admits that often she has been "giving in." She reports it has been years since she last saw a dentist and eye doctor, due to the lack of free or sliding-scale providers for uninsured patients and long waiting lists.

You finally speak with Maria on the phone today, just before she leaves for work at 5 p.m. However, she can't speak with you long, as she has to leave early to make multiple stops to pick up her youngest child from daycare before grabbing dinner for them. She explains that she couldn't attend the last appointment because she had to take her groceries home first and needed to make dinner once she arrived home an hour later because she didn't want her kids to eat KFC for another night during the week (Maria also reports that each time she does that, she spends $20). She often gets ideas about what to eat from the billboards she sees on her way home on the bus. The main reason why she can't return to the clinic to follow up on the Pap test result is that "I can't take time off from work. I work the night shift and sleep when the clinic is open." Moreover, Maria expresses some reluctance to find out a diagnosis, as she worries what relational problems this may raise. Not only is she afraid of finding out that she may have cancer, but she says she's heard different things about causes of cervical cancer, and she's worried about being "embarrassed" by what people might think of her if she is diagnosed with cervical cancer.

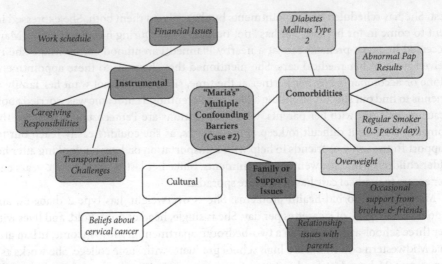

Figure 1.4 Maria's stressors and barriers.

What possible multidisciplinary interventions would be important for Maria (Figure 1.4)?

- Educate Maria about prevention and some of the known risk factors for cervical cancer, breast cancer, diabetes, and other diseases (e.g., diet/nutrition, exercise, preventive cancer screenings, smoking)
- Schedule diagnostic test
- Lifestyle modifications
- Address barriers to care: scheduling barriers, cost of losing working hours, transportation difficulty, childcare responsibilities, patient's denial/anxiety/ambivalence about diagnosis.

Poverty Profiles of Low-Income Women

Since there are also unique needs of subpopulations of low-income women of color living in urban areas, we will next describe a range of poverty profiles—female head of household with children, 65-plus years old, the working poor, rural residents, homeless women, those who are temporarily poor, those who are chronically poor, and racial minorities—and the barriers that each category of women encounters. We list common concerns we have heard low-income women report and have developed a list of "if/then" statements providers can use to respond to these problems. We provide real-life examples of stressors that these women report, such as financial strain in meeting basic necessities, being unemployed or having work demands, housing challenges, untreated mental/emotional issues, addiction, legal issues, caregiving demands, trauma related to experiencing violence and loss, other illness or disability, and mistreatment by healthcare providers. We hope that these examples can be used to teach providers about the types of stressors and barriers they will help these women try to address.

Female Head of Household with Children

Women in this category can be described as being divorced or never married and may not receive child support. In 2017, those households maintained by women with no husband present had the lowest median income ($41,909), compared to married-couple households ($88,929) and households maintained by men with no wife present ($59,299) (Fontenot et al., 2018). For related children in families with a female head of household, 40.8% were in poverty, compared with 8.4% of related children in married-couple families (Fontenot et al., 2018). Between 2016 and 2017, it was reported that one in four women had trouble paying medical bills, using most of their savings or borrowed money; as a result, many delayed receiving care (Borchelt, 2018). Many women have dead-end jobs with hourly wages, no security, and no room for advancement. These jobs tend to pay less.

Across the United States, average costs for childcare exceed 27% of median household income for single working parents, with even higher rates for families of color (Child Care Aware of America, 2018). Hence, childcare costs lead to difficult choices about employment and deployment of family resources for many low-income parents (Davis et al., 2018b).

Financial/Medical Insurance Concerns
If . . .

- I don't have medical insurance.
- I don't have money because I have bills to pay.
- I can't afford the co-pay.
- I can't even put food on the table.

Then . . .

- I can find out if you are eligible to receive a free or low-cost screening. For example, we can consider resources such as FQHCs, local mammogram van programs, or Planned Parenthood.

Transportation
If . . .

- I don't have money to get there.
- I don't have a car or a ride.
- I don't drive.
- I don't have anyone to take me.

Then . . .

- I can help you determine the bus or train you need to take. I can get the telephone number and websites for the public transport line and bus lines near your area. I can help provide a taxi voucher. I can help connect you to local transportation assistance programs.

Caregiving, Childcare, and Safety Issues
If . . .

- I've got to take care of my kids.
- I need childcare.

Then . . .

- I can refer you to some low-cost childcare resources that can help you.
- I can find out if the clinic has a play area or someone on site who watches children during appointments.

Work Demands
If . . .

- I work the night shift, and I'm asleep when the clinic is open.
- I can't take off from work.
- I work Monday through Friday.
- I need to find work.

Then . . .

- I can find a time that works at a clinic that has evening and Saturday hours.

Health Not a Priority
If . . .

- I can't even put food on the table; why should I care about cancer?
- What difference does a screening make? It won't make me not have cancer if I already have it.

Then . . .

- Your health and ability to care for your family affects your ability to put food on the table.
- By getting screened, you can know what you are dealing with and you can make decisions about what will work for you to stay healthy.

Competing Time/Scheduling Priorities
If . . .

- I just don't have time. All the time I get off from work, I try to spend with my kids.
- My kids stay with friends; I have to go by their schedule.

Then . . .

- I can find a time that works at a clinic that has evening and Saturday hours.

65-Plus Years Old

Women in this category often have a lack of income and few assets. They may rely on their Social Security income. They often experience rising expenses, high medical costs, and failing health.

Transportation

If . . .

- I don't have a car or a way to get there.
- I am not physically able to take public transportation.

Then . . .

- I can help you determine the bus or train you need to take. For example, I can get the telephone number and websites for the public transport line and bus lines near your area. I can help you order a taxi or offer a voucher. I can help connect you with local transportation assistance programs.

Physical Limitations

If . . .

- I am hard of hearing and can't go by myself.

Then . . .

- Let's discuss a close family member or friend who can accompany you. Who might be able to help? What is their relationship to you? How do you plan to contact them?

Proximity Concerns

If . . .

- The clinic is too far away.
- I will have to walk too far to catch the bus.
- The clinic is in a bad area.

Then . . .

- We can get a taxi to pick you up at your house.
- We can call the clinic to have someone meet you at the door.

Financial/Medical Insurance Concerns

If . . .

- I can't afford the co-pay.
- I'm on a fixed income.
- Medicare doesn't cover that.

Then . . .

- I can find out if you are eligible to receive a free or low-cost screening. For example, we can check availability of screenings at an FQHC or a Planned Parenthood clinic.

Caregiving
If . . .

- I can't leave my spouse.
- I can't leave my grandkids alone.

Then . . .

- Let's discuss if you have another family member to watch them.
- Let's look into any child or adult daycare resources that might be possible.

Health Not a Priority
If . . .

- I'm too old to worry about cancer.

Then . . .

- You are never too old to worry about your health, and staying healthy for as long as possible for your loved ones should be important.

Feelings of Discrimination
If . . .

- Doctors discriminate against the elderly.

Then . . .

- We can refer you to a different doctor or a different clinic.

Education/Literacy Problems
If . . .

- I have trouble filling out forms on my own.
- I don't know what to ask the doctor.

Then . . .

- We can start by going over the things you don't understand over the phone and then you can follow up with a case manager or social worker at the clinic who can further assist you with the forms.

Working Poor

Women in the working poor demographic are those who are working in the service sector and work long or inconvenient hours (night shifts). Jobs pay low wages and women often work only parttime, and not by choice. These women make too much money for government support but too little money to support a family. They constantly live in fear of losing the job they have.

Work Demands
If . . .

- I can't take time off from work.
- I work the night shift and sleep when the clinic is open.
- I only work during the summer, so I have to work now and save for winter. I'll go then.
- I work Monday through Friday.
- I don't have a replacement if I take time off from work.
- I have a new job and I am on probation; I can't take off now.

Then . . .

- I can find a time that works at a clinic that has evening and Saturday hours.

Financial/Medical Insurance Concerns
If . . .

- I don't have insurance.
- I can't afford it.
- I can't even put food on the table.

Then . . .

- I can find out if you are eligible to receive a free or low-cost screening. For example, we can check if there are any FQHCs, local mammogram vans, or Planned Parenthood sites that may be helpful.

Transportation
If . . .

- I can't afford the bus and I don't have a car.

Then . . .

- I can find out if you are eligible to receive free transportation.
- I can help you determine the bus or train you need to take. For example, I can get the telephone number and websites for the public transport line and bus lines in your area.
- I can help you get a taxi and offer a voucher to help you get to your appointment.

Employment Uncertainties
If . . .

- I might lose my job any time.

Then . . .

- We don't want you to lose your job. We can help find a clinic that has late or Saturday hours.

Rural Residents

These women have fewer job opportunities, and those that exist pay low wages. They lack transportation. Fewer social services (healthcare, childcare, and education) are available, and they are of lower quality.

Proximity Concerns
If . . .

- There's no clinic near me.

Then . . .

- I can find out if there is a mobile screening van coming to your area.

Shame
If . . .

- I don't want people to see me going to the clinic. This is a small town.

Then . . .

- I can understand wanting to keep some things private. I will help you look for a feasible alternative location.

Financial
If . . .

- I can't afford it.

Then . . .

- I can find out if you are eligible to receive free screenings.

Transportation
If . . .

- I don't have a car, and there's no public transportation.

Then...

- I can find out if you are eligible to receive free or low-cost transportation.

Work Demands
If...

- I can't take time off work or they'll fire me.

Then...

- I can find a clinic that offers late or Saturday hours.

Homeless Women

Homeless women find it difficult to obtain and maintain jobs. The shelters where they stay may not be safe. They may also be caring for children and/or leaving abusive relationships. These women may also have a mental illness.

Shelter
If...

- Right now I'm only worried about finding a place to stay.

Then...

- I can get in contact with 2-1-1 to find you help in getting a place to stay. I can help connect you with 2-1-1 operators, and offer you a list of 2-1-1 shelters.

Financial
If...

- I can't afford it.

Then...

- I can find out if you are eligible for free or low-cost services.
- Most FQHCs will not turn anyone away based on ability to pay, and offer sliding-scale fees with payments as low as $10 or programs to help.

No Address/Telephone
If...

- There's no way for the doctor to contact me even if I do go. I'll never know the results, so why bother?

Then...

- Is there an alternative way to contact you? Is there a friend, neighbor, social worker, or church with whom we can leave a message?

Health Not a Priority
If . . .

- I've got bigger things to worry about than cancer right now.

Then . . .

- If you take care of your health, it could be one less thing you have to worry about.

Transportation
If . . .

- I don't have a way to get there.

Then . . .

- I can find out if you are eligible to receive free transportation.
- I can help you determine the bus or train you need to take. For example, I can get the telephone number and websites for the public transport line and bus lines near your area.
- I can arrange a taxi to pick you up and offer a voucher to pay.

Childcare/Safety Issues
If . . .

- I can't leave my kids or my abusive partner might find them.

Then . . .

- I can get work with 2-1-1 to find you help. I can connect you with 2-1-1 operators and offer you a list of emergency shelters.

Healthcare System Issues
If . . .

- There are always long waits.
- That clinic is always so crowded and busy.

Then . . .

- I can call the clinic to see what their schedule looks like on the days you are available to go. (Tuesdays and Fridays are usually slower days at clinics, but services vary on certain days. Check with the individual clinics for specific schedules.)

Experience with Poor Customer Relations
If . . .

- They don't treat me well at the clinics.
- The staff is unprofessional.

Then . . .

- If you are having a problem with a particular clinic, I can schedule you at a different one.
- I can find out who you can talk to at the clinic if you have a complaint. Each clinic has a suggestion or complaint box. Information on how to file a formal complaint is contained in the Patient Bill of Rights posted at each clinic.

Temporary Poverty

During the four-year period from 2009 to 2012, 34.5% of the population had at least one spell of poverty lasting two or more months (Fontenot et al., 2018, 21). Between the ages of 25 to 60, 61.8% of the population will experience a year below the 20th percentile, and 42.1% will experience a year below the 10th percentile (Rank & Hirschl, 2015). Many of these women may have recently lost their job and are quickly searching for another.

Financial
If . . .

- I'll just wait until I get a job with insurance.
- I'm too busy looking for a job.

Then . . .

- I can help you find a clinic that is on a sliding-fee scale or one where no insurance is needed.

Transportation
If . . .

- I can't afford the gas to get there right now.

Then . . .

- I can find out if you are eligible to receive free or low-cost transportation.
- I can help you figure out the bus/train to take to get to the clinic. For example, I can get the telephone number and websites for the public transport line and bus lines near your area.
- I can help arrange a taxi to transport you and offer a voucher to pay.

Childcare
If . . .

- I can't find anyone to watch my kids.

Then . . .

- I can find a time that works for you.
- I can find out if you can bring your children with you to the appointment.

Chronic Poverty

This group comprises only 10% to 15% of poor Americans. They usually have characteristics that put them at a disadvantage in the labor market, such as disabilities, single-parent families with many children, and minorities in poor job markets.

Transportation
If . . .

- I can't afford the bus/train.

Then . . .

- I can find out if you are eligible to receive free or low-cost transportation.

Caretaking/Childcare Issues
If . . .

- I can't find anyone to watch my kids.

Then . . .

- I can find out if you can bring your children with you to the appointment.

Literacy Issues
If . . .

- I have trouble filling out forms.
- I don't know what to ask the doctor.

Then . . .

- Do you have anyone you can bring with you to the appointment to help you?
- I can find out if there is someone at the clinic who can help you with forms.

Lack of Employment/Limited Employment
If . . .

- I'm too busy looking for a job.

Then . . .

- We can talk about your schedule and find a time that works for you.

Experience with Poor Customer Relations
If . . .

- They don't treat me well at the clinics.

Then...

- If you are having a problem with a particular clinic, I can schedule you at a different one.
- I can find out who you can talk to at the clinic if you have a complaint. Most clinics have a suggestion or complaint box on the premises. Procedures for how to file a formal complaint are contained in the Patient Bill of Rights posted at each location.

Racial/Ethnic Minorities or "Underclass"

Minorities face discrimination and lack of opportunities. There are differences in family structure (e.g., more single-parent families).

Experience with Poor Customer Relations

If...

- I don't go to that hospital/clinic because they are racist. The doctors discriminate against me!
- The staff at the clinics don't know how to treat people.

Then...

- If you are treated badly, I can help you find the information you need to report the clinic staff.
- I can schedule you at a different clinic.

Different Social/Religious Customs and Citizenship Status

If...

- Because of my religion, I can't see a male doctor.
- I'm not a U.S. citizen and I'm afraid of being reported if I go to the clinic.
- There's not much people can do to lower their chances of getting cancer; if God wants me to get it, it will happen regardless of if I get a screening.

Then...

- I can find out if the clinic has a female doctor or nurse who is available.
- The clinics are able to treat you even though you are not a U.S. citizen. and they do not report your status to authorities.
- Yes, this is true; but it has been shown that screening increases the chances of detecting certain cancers early, when they are most likely to be curable.

Literacy Issues/Trouble Navigating the System

If...

- I have trouble filling out forms.
- I don't know what to ask the doctor.
- I don't know anything about a mammogram/Pap test/colonoscopy, etc.
- I feel fine now. I don't need to go to the doctor.

Then . . .

- Do you have anyone you can bring with you to the appointment to help you? If not, I can find out if there is someone at the clinic who can help you with forms.
- I can help you with questions to ask the doctor.
- I can explain the procedure and/or what happens during the screening; I can also provide you with information from the National Cancer Institute website and cancer fact sheets.
- Sometimes breast cancer has no obvious symptoms at all.

References

Ashing-Giwa, K. T. (1999). Quality of life and psychosocial outcomes in long-term survivors of breast cancer: A focus on African American women. *Journal of Psychosocial Oncology, 17*(3/4), 47–62.

Ashing-Giwa, K. T., Padilla, G., Tejero, J., Kraemer, J., Wright, K., Coscarelli, A., Clayton, S., Williams, I., & Hills, D. (2004). Understanding the breast cancer experience of women: A qualitative study of African American, Asian American, Latina and Caucasian cancer survivors. *Psycho-Oncology, 13*, 408–428.

Baker, J. L., & Jemmott, L. S. (2014). The role of environmental context, faith, and patient satisfaction in HIV prevention among African American women. *Journal of Obstetric, Gynecologic, and Neonatal Nursing, 43*(5), 631–632. https://doi.org/10.1111/1552-6909.12490

Banegas, M. P., Dickerson, J. F., Kent, E. E., de Moor, J. S., Virgo, K. S., Guy, G. P., Jr, Ekwueme, D. U., Zheng, Z., Nutt, S., Pace, L., Varga, A., Waiwaiole, L., Schneider, J., & Robin Yabroff, K. (2018). Exploring barriers to the receipt of necessary medical care among cancer survivors under age 65 years. *Journal of Cancer Survivorship: Research and Practice, 12*(1), 28–37. https://doi.org/10.1007/s11764-017-0640-1

Beckjord, E. B., & Klassen, A. C. (2008). Cultural values and secondary prevention of breast cancer in African American women. *Cancer Control, 15*(1), 63–71.

Bernard, V., Howe, W., Royalty, J., Helsel, W., Kammerer, W., & Richardson, L. (2012). Timeliness of cervical cancer diagnosis and initiation of treatment in the Nation Breast and Cervical Cancer Early Detection Program. *Journal of Women's Health, 21*, 776–782.

Borchelt, G. (2018). The impact poverty has on women's health. *Human Rights, 43*(3), 16–19.

Bourjolly, J. N. (1998). Differences in religiousness among Black and White women with breast cancer. *Social Work in Health Care, 28*(1), 21–39.

Bourjolly, J. N., & Hirschman, K. B. (2001). Similarities in coping strategies but differences in sources of support among African American and White women coping with breast cancer. *Journal of Psychosocial Oncology, 19*(2), 17–38.

Bradley, P. K. (2005). The delay and worry experience of African American women with breast cancer. *Oncology Nursing Forum, 32*(2), 243–249.

Caplan, L. S., & Helzlsouer, K. J. (1992–93). Delay in breast cancer: A review of the literature. *Public Health Reviews, 20*(3-4), 187–214.

Child Care Aware of America. (2018). *The US and the high cost of child care: A review of prices and proposed solutions for a broken system: 2018 report.* https://www.childcareaware.org/our-issues/research/the-us-and-the-high-price-of-child-care-2019/

Cofie, L. E., Hirth, J. M., & Wong, R. (2018). Chronic comorbidities and cervical cancer screening and adherence among US-born and foreign-born women. *Cancer Causes & Control, 29,* 1105–1113.

Copeland, V. C., Scholle, S. H., & Binko, J. A. (2003). Patient satisfaction: African American women's views of the patient–doctor relationship. *Journal of Health & Social Policy, 17*(2), 35–48.

Culver, J. L., Arena, P. L., Antoni, M. H., & Carver, C. S. (2002). Coping and distress among women under treatment for early stage breast cancer: Comparing African Americans, Hispanics and non-Hispanic Whites. *Psycho-Oncology, 11,* 495–504.

Davey, M. P., Bilkins, B., Diamond, G., Willis, A. I., Mitchell, E. P., Davey, A., & Young, F. M. (2016). African American patients' psychosocial support needs and barriers to treatment: Patient needs assessment. *Journal of Cancer Education, 31,* 481–487.

Davis, C. M., Nyamathi, A. M., Abuatiq, A., Fike, G. C., & Wilson, A. M. (2016). Understanding supportive care factors among African American breast cancer survivors. *Journal of Transcultural Nursing, 29*(1), 21–29. doi:10.1177/1043659616670713

Davis, E. E., Carlin, C., Krafft, C., & Forry, N. D. (2018b). Do child care subsidies increase employment among low-income parents? *Journal of Family and Economic Issues, 39,* 662–682.

Ell, K., Quon, B., Quinn, D. I., Dwight-Johnson, M., Wells, A., & Lee, P. (2007). Improving treatment of depression among low-income patients with cancer: The design of the ADAPt-C study. *General Hospital Psychiatry, 29,* 223–231.

Flannery, I. M., Yoo, G. J., & Levine, E. G. (2019). Keeping us all whole: Acknowledging the agency of African American breast cancer survivors and their systems of social support. *Supportive Care in Cancer, 27*(7), 2625–2632. https://doi.org/10.1007/s00520-018-4538-x

Fontenot, K., Semega, J., & Kollar, M. (2017). Income and poverty in the United States: 2017. U.S. Census Bureau. https://www.census.gov/library/publications/2018/demo/p60-263.html

Fowler, B. A. (2006). Claiming health: Mammography screening decision making of African American women. *Oncology Nursing Forum, 33*(5), 969–975.

Gibson, L. M., & Hendricks, C. S. (2006). Integrative review of spirituality in African American breast cancer survivors. *ABNF Journal, 17*(2), 67–72.

Gullate, M. (2006). The influence of spirituality and religiosity on breast cancer screening delay in African American women: Application of the Theory of Reasoned Action and Planned Behavior (TRA/TPB). *ABNF Journal, 17,* 89–94.

Gullatte, M. M., Brawley, O., Kinney, A., Powe, B., & Mooney, K. (2010). Religiosity, spirituality, and cancer fatalism beliefs on delay in breast cancer diagnosis in African American women. *Journal of Religion and Health, 49*(1), 62–72. https://doi.org/10.1007/s10943-008-9232-8

Henderson, P. D., Gore, S. V., Davis, B. L., & Condon, E. H. (2003). African American women coping with breast cancer: A qualitative analysis. *Oncology Nursing Forum, 30*(4), 641–647.

Holt, C. L., Kyles, A., Wiehagen, T., & Casey, C. (2003a). Development of a spiritually based breast cancer education booklet for African American women. *Cancer Control, 10*(5), 37–44.

Holt, C. L., Lukwago, S. N., & Kreuter, M. (2003b). Spirituality, breast cancer beliefs and mammography utilization among urban African American women. *Journal of Health Psychology, 8*(3), 383–396.

Horner, M. J., Alterkruse, S. F., Zou, Z., Wideroff, L., Katki, H. A., & Stinchcomb, D. G. (2011). U.S. geographic distribution of prevaccine era cervical cancer screening, incidence, stage, and mortality. *Cancer Epidemiology & Biomarkers, 20,* 591–599.

Jones, D. P. (2015). Knowledge, beliefs and feelings about breast cancer: The perspective of African American women. *ABNF Journal*, *26*(1), 5–10.

Klassen, A. C., & Washington, C. (2008). How does social integration influence breast cancer control among urban African-American women? Results from a cross-sectional survey. *BMC Women's Health*, *8*, 4. https://doi.org/10.1186/1472-6874-8-4

Krok-Schoen, J. L., Oliveri, J. M., Young, G. S., Katz, M. L., Tatum, C. M., & Paskett, E. D. (2016). Evaluating the stage of change model to a cervical cancer screening intervention among Ohio Appalachian women. *Women & Health*, *56*(4), 468–486.

Lang, M. J., Giese-Davis, J., Patton, S. B., & Campbell, D. J. T. (2018). Does age matter? Comparing post-treatment psychosocial outcomes in young adult and older adult cancer survivors with their cancer-free peers. *Psycho-Oncology*, *27*(1), 1404–1411.

Lynn, B., Yoo, G. J., & Levine, E. G. (2014). "Trust in the Lord": Religious and spiritual practices of African American breast cancer survivors. *Journal of Religion and Health*, *53*(6), 1706–1716. https://doi.org/10.1007/s10943-013-9750-x

Marouf, A., Mortada, H., & Fakiha, M. G. (2020). Psychological, sociodemographic, and clinicopathological predictors of breast cancer patients' decision to undergo breast reconstruction after mastectomy. *Saudi Medical Journal*, *41*(3), 267–274. https://doi.org/10.15537/smj.2020.3.24946

McDaniel, J. S., Musselman, D. L., Porter, M. R., Reed, D. A., & Nemeroff, C. B. (1995). Depression in patients with cancer: Diagnosis, biology, and treatment. *Archives of General Psychiatry*, *52*, 89–99.

McDonald, P. A., Thorne, D. D., Pearson, J. C., & Adams-Campbell, L. L. (1999, Winter), Perceptions and knowledge of breast cancer among African American women residing in public housing. *Ethnicity & Disease*, *9*(1), 81–93.

Meichenbaum, D., & Turk, D.C. (1987). *Facilitating treatment adherence*. Plenum Press.

Meyerowitz, B. E., Formenti, S. C., Ell, K. O., & Leedham, B. (2000). Depression among Latina cervical cancer patients. *Journal of Social and Clinical Psychology*, *19*(3), 352–371.

Misra-Herbert, A. D. (2017). Cervical cancer in African American women: Optimizing prevention to reduce disparities. *Cleveland Clinic Journal of Medicine*, *84*(10), 795–796.

Mitchell, J., Lannin, D. R., Mathews, H. F., & Swanson, M. S. (2002). Religious beliefs and breast cancer screening. *Journal of Women's Health*, *11*(10), 907–915.

Morgan, P., Barnett, K., Perdue, B., Fogel, J., Underwood, S. M., Gaskins, M., & Brown-Davis, C. (2006, January/February). African American women with breast cancer and their spouses' perception of care received from physicians. *ABNF Journal*, *17*(1), 32–37.

Morgan, P., Fogel, J., Rose, L., Barnett, K., Mock, V., Davis, B. L., Gaskins, M., & Brown-Davis, C. (2005). African American couples merging strengths to successfully cope with breast cancer. *Oncology Nursing Forum*, *32*(5), 979–987.

Morgan, S. E., Occa, A., Potter, J., Mouton, A., & Peter, M. E. (2017). "You need to be a good listener": Recruiter's use of relational communication behaviors to enhance clinical trial and research study accrual. *Journal of Health Communication*, *22*, 95–101.

Nickell, A., Stewart, S. L., Burke, N. J., Guerra, C., Cohen, E., Lawlor, C., Colen, S., Cheng, J., & Joseph, G. (2019). Engaging limited English proficient and ethnically diverse low-income women in health research: A randomized trial of a patient navigator intervention. *Patient Education and Counseling*, *102*, 1313–1323.

Nonzee, N. J., Ragas, D. M., Ha Luu, T., Phisuthikul, A. M., Tom, L., Dong, X., & Simon, M. A. (2015). Delays in cancer care among low-income minorities despite access. *Journal of Women's Health*, *24*(6), 506–514. https://doi.org/10.1089/jwh.2014.4998

Ogle, K. S., Swanson, G. M., Woods, N., & Azzouz, F. (2000). Cancer and comorbidity: Redefining chronic diseases. *Cancer, 88*(3), 653–663. doi:10.1002/(SICI)1097 0142(20000201)88:3<653::AID-CNCR24>3.0.CO;2-1.

Paladino, A. J., Anderson, J. N., Krukowski, R. A., Waters, T., Kocak, M., Graff, C., Blue, R., Jones, T. N., Buzaglo, J., Vidal, G., Pasick, R., & Burke, N. J. (2008). A critical review of theory in breast cancer screening promotion across cultures. *Annual Review of Public Health, 29*, 351–368. https://doi.org/10.1146/annurey.publhealth.29.020907.143420

Pasick, R. J., & Burke, N. J. (2008). A critical review of theory in breast cancer screening promotion across cultures. *Annual Review of Public Health, 29*(1), 351–368. https://doi.org/10.1146/annurev.publhealth.29.020907.143420

Paterniti, D. A., Melnikow, J., Nuovo, J., Henderson, S., DeGregorio, M., Kuppermann, M., & Nease, R. (2005). "I'm going to die of something anyway": Women's perceptions of tamoxifen for breast cancer risk reduction. *Ethnicity & Disease, 15*(3), 365–372.

Pullen, E., Perry, B., & Oser, C. (2014). African American women's preventative care usage: The role of social support and racial experiences and attitudes. *Sociology of Health & Illness, 36*(7), 1037–1053. https://doi.org/10.1111/1467-9566.12141

Rank, M. R., & Hirschl, T. A. (2015). The likelihood of experiencing relative poverty over the life course. *PLoS One, 10*(7), e0133513. doi:10.1371/journal.pone.0133514)

Rice, W. S., Logie, C. H., Napoles, T. M., Walcott, M., Batchelder, A. W., Kempf, M., Wingood, G. M., Konkle-Parker, D. J., Turan, B., Wilson, T. E., O'Johnson, M., Weiser, S. D., & Turan, J.M. (2018). Perceptions of intersectional stigma among diverse women living with HIV in the United States. *Social Science & Medicine, 208*, 9–17.

Richardson, J. L., & Sanchez, K. (1998). Compliance with cancer treatment. In J. C. Holland (Ed.), *Psycho-oncology*. Oxford University Press, 67–77.

Richardson Gibson, L. M., & Parker, V. (2003). Inner resources as predictors of psychological well-being in middle-income African American breast cancer survivors. *Cancer Control, 10*(5), 52–59. https://doi.org/10.1177/107327480301005s08

Rodriguez, A. (2017). Addressing social determinant factors that negatively impact an individual's health. AJMC Managed Markets and Network. https://www.ajmc.com/newsroom/social-determinant-factors-can-negatively-impact-an-individuals-health

Rumun, A. J. (2014). Influence of religious beliefs on healthcare practice. *International Journal of Education and Research, 2*, 37–48.

Sage, S. K., Hawkins-Taylor, C., Crockett, R. A., Sr, & Balls-Berry, J. E. (2020). "Girl, just pray . . .": Factors that influence breast and cervical cancer screening among Black women in Rochester, MN. *Journal of the National Medical Association, 112*(5), 454–467. https://doi.org/10.1016/j.jnma.2019.02.006

Schulz, E., Holt, C. L., Caplan, L., Blake, V., Southward, P., Buckner, A., & Lawrence, H. (2008). Role of spirituality in cancer coping among African Americans: A qualitative examination. *Journal of Cancer Survivorship: Research and Practice, 2*(2), 104–115. https://doi.org/10.1007/s11764-008-0050-5

Schwartzberg, L., & Graetz, I. (2019). THRIVE study protocol: A randomized controlled trial evaluating a web-based app and tailored messages to improve adherence to adjuvant endocrine therapy among women with breast cancer. *BMC Health Services Research, 19*(1), 977. https://doi.org/10.1186/s12913-019-4588-x

Selove, R., Kilbourne, B., Fadden, M. K., Sanderson, M., Foster, M., Offodile, R., Husaini, B., Mouton, C., & Levine, R. S. (2016). Time from screening mammography to biopsy and from biopsy to breast cancer treatment among Black and White, women Medicare beneficiaries not participating in a health maintenance organization. *Sexual & Reproductive Health*, *26*(6), 642–647. https://doi.org/10.1016/j.whi.2016.09.003

Sheppard, J. P., Stevens, S., Stevens, R., Martin, U., Mant, J., Hobbs, F. D., & McManus, R. J. (2018). Benefits and harms of antihypertensive treatment in low-risk patients with mild hypertension. *JAMA Internal Medicine*, *178*(12), 1626–1634. doi:10.1001/jamainternmed.2018.4684

Sohn, H. (2017). Racial and ethnic disparities in health insurance coverage: Dynamics of gaining and losing coverage over the life-course. *Population Research and Policy Review*, *36*(2), 181–201. doi:10.1007/s11113-016-9416-y

Stevens, A., Courtney-Long, E., Gillespie, C., & Armour, B. S. (2014). Hypertension among US adults by disability status and type, National Health and Nutrition Examination Survey, 2001–2010. *Preventing Chronic Disease*, *11*, E139.

Talley, C. H., Yang, L., & Williams, K. P. (2017). Breast cancer screening paved with good intentions: Application of the information–motivation–behavioral skills model to racial/ethnic minority women. *Journal of Immigrant and Minority Health*, *19*(6), 1362–1371. https://doi.org/10.1007/s10903-016-0355-9

Tejeda, S., Darnell, J. S., Cho, Y. I., Stolley, M. R., Markossian, T. W., & Calhoun, E. A. (2013). Patient barriers to follow-up care for breast and cervical cancer abnormalities. *Journal of Women's Health*, *22*(6), 507–517.

Turner, R. J., & Avison, W. R. (2003). Status variations in stress exposure: Implications for the interpretation of research on race, socioeconomic status, and gender. *Journal of Health and Social Behavior*, *44*, 488–505.

Villa, M. L., Cuellar, J., Gamel, N., & Yeo, G. (1993). *Aging and health: Hispanic American elders* (2nd edition). SGEC Working Paper Series, Number 5, Ethnogeriatric Reviews, Stanford Geriatric Education Center.

Wallner, L. P., McLeod, C., Hamilton, A. S., Ward, K. C., Veenstra, C. M., An, L. C., Janz, N. K., Katz, S. J., & Hawley, S. T. (2017). Decision-support networks of women newly diagnosed with breast cancer. *Cancer*, *123*(20), 3895–3903. https://doi.org/10.1002/cncr.30848

Wang, J. H., Mandelblatt, J. S., Liang, W., Yi, B., Ma, I. J., & Schwartz, M. D. (2009). Knowledge, cultural, and attitudinal barriers to mammography screening among nonadherent immigrant Chinese women: Ever versus never screened status. *Cancer*, *115*(20), 4828–4838. https://doi.org/10.1002/cncr.24517

Warren-Findlow, J., & Prohaska, T. R. (2008). Families, social support, and self-care among older African American women with chronic illness. *American Journal of Health Promotion*, *22*(5), 342–349.

Weil, E., Wachterman, M., McCarthy, E. P., Davis, R. B., O'Day, B., Iezzoni, L. I., & Wee, C. C. (2002). Obesity among adults with disabling conditions. *Journal of the American Medical Association*, *288*, 1265–1268.

Wells, A., Palinkas, L., Williams, S., & Ell, K. (2014). Retaining low-income minority cancer patients to depression treatment intervention trial: Lessons learned. *Community Mental Health Journal*, *51*(6), 715–722. doi:10.1007/s10597-014-9819-3

Wells, A., Sanders Thompson, V. L., Camp Yeakey, C., & Notaro, S. (2019). *Poverty and place: Cancer prevention among low-income women of color*. Lexington Books.

Wells, N. L., & Turney, M. E. (2001). Common issues facing adults with cancer. In M. M. Lauria, E. J. Clark, J. F. Hermann, & N. M. Stearns (Eds.), *Social work in oncology*. American Cancer Society, 27–44.

Whyte, L. W. (2000). Promoting health prevention programs and medical compliance: An expanded conceptual model. In S. L. Logan & E. M. Freeman (Eds.), *Health care in the black community*. Haworth Press, 83–95.

Wilmoth, M. C., & Sanders, L. D. (2001). Accept me for myself: African American women's issues after breast cancer. *Oncology Nursing Forum, 28*(5), 875–879.

Young, T., & Maher, J. (1999). Collecting quality of life data in EORTC clinical trials—what happens in practice? *Psycho-Oncology, 8*(3), 260–263.

Module 1.3: Culturally Competent Communication, Assessment, and Engagement

Health cannot be a question of income; it is a fundamental human right.
Nelson Mandela (December 2003)

In this module we discuss the relevance and importance of cultural competency in communication, assessment, and engagement with our patients. Particularly with practice among low-income women of color, their lived experiences are descriptors of intersectionality. For this reason, we must we first be aware of, accepting of, and knowledgeable about difference. In this section, we discuss not only diverse racial/ethnic and socioeconomic populations but also patient populations characterized by a variety of religious affiliations. By no means does this discussion capture all populations of low-income women of color, as there is diversity based on gender, age, sexual orientation, disability, immigration status, and other important characteristics and identifications.

Culturally competent practice is essential for the successful implementation of any intervention. Use of the expanded CCM must be combined with cultural competence at every level. We cannot understand the importance of cultural competence without first discussing the concept of culture. Culture is identified as one's worldview that includes "experiences, expressions, symbols, materials, customs, behaviors, morals, values, attitudes, and beliefs created and communicated among individuals" (Villa et al., 1993)—but it goes deeper than that. Culture actually includes all the elements that make us unique. It influences our relationships, ideas, and how we choose to live our life. We can think of culture with respect to a common ethnic or religious heritage that was passed on to us from our parents and grandparents. We can also consider the culture within the hospital or clinic where we work—for instance, the values and beliefs of the helping profession that we share and the communication we use when speaking to colleagues or documenting about our patients.

Cultural values and beliefs represent a shared way of thinking, behaving, and viewing the world. For example, in many Asian ethnic groups (such as Chinese, Japanese, and Koreans), cultural values and beliefs include filial piety, deference to authority, and the importance of saving face (Iwamoto & Liu, 2010; Lum, 2011). Some cultures do not value education because it is not seen historically as a means to succeed or to escape poverty. Here we see that cultural beliefs are often influenced by the context in which the individual lives.

What Is Cultural Competency?

Various definitions of cultural competence have been offered through decades of scholarship in healthcare, social sciences, and other fields of study and practice. According to one definition,

> Cultural competence is a continuous learning process that builds knowledge, awareness, skills and capacity to identify, understand and respect the unique beliefs, values, customs, language, abilities and traditions of all, in order to develop policies to promote effective programs and services. (Ohio Mental Health and Addiction Services, 2016)

This is a comprehensive definition that includes both the healthcare provider and the patient. It's important to understand that both the provider and the patient can understand and appreciate cultures and belief systems other than their own, and this is critical to adherence and the helping process.

Five dimensions of a culturally competent practitioner have been proposed:

1. Awareness and acceptance of difference
2. Cultural self-awareness
3. Understanding the dynamics of difference
4. Developing cultural knowledge
5. Adaptation of practice skills to fit the cultural context of the client (Cross et al., 1989).

While the goal of this module is to focus on "adaptation of practice skills" in cancer care among low-income women of color, this also requires some discussion of the four preceding dimensions. As such, this section will seek to promote awareness and knowledge of some of the practice skills relevant to populations of low-income women of color.

Why Is Cultural Competency Important to the Practice with Low-Income Women of Color?

Cultural competency is a necessary part of the helping relationship and can occur at every phase of the cancer continuum. Those working in cancer care with low-income women of color must become culturally competent. This means understanding that every woman is unique and that every woman is from a diverse background and experience. The idea of a "one-size-fits-all" solution does not account for the intersections of race and culture and can lead to disparities across all systems. Sometimes hasty decisions and first impressions are used to understand and make meaning, but they might not be accurate. Providers should take an individualized approach to meeting the unique needs of each woman and can also help reconcile personal barriers and challenges. Don't assume that what works for one woman will also work for another woman with a similar profile. Through discussions with other healthcare providers, you will gain new insight and ideas in working with diverse communities. Healthcare providers who are culturally competent and have orientations toward diversity generally tend to be able not only to tease out subtle biases but also promote better adherence among women.

Cultural competency can be challenging in an interdisciplinary setting comprising different provider disciplines and different patient backgrounds, all of which involve different values, health beliefs, and preferences. These differences often explain why some women opt for chemotherapy or radiation or others believe that radiation causes cancer and opt for noninvasive treatments. When providers and women better understand each other's respective illness representations, they are better able to reconcile differences in viewpoints and come to agreement with options for preventive screening or treatment regimens. When this happens, women are better able to solve problems, make informed decisions, feel empowered, and have more trust in their healthcare providers and the healthcare system. This can contribute to better health directly by lowering apprehension and improving the woman's commitment to cancer prevention or treatment recommendations.

Cultural Competency in Practice

Cultural competence starts with being a good listener, which means stop talking and just actively listen. Listening goes a long way in understanding the needs of women and the communities we practice in. Active listening can take the form of starting a conversation to elicit insight and understanding. While we are actively listening, it is important to try to be empathetic, which means not being afraid to "walk in their shoes." By showing non-judgmental attentiveness, avoiding interruption, asking about the patient's beliefs and values, and giving clinical information in a way the patient understands, we communicate our commitment, respect, and interest in the patient as a person. In turn, when patients share their beliefs, values, and preferences, they are sharing information that provides opportunities for us to understand them better and for both parties to discover common ground.

As a healthcare provider, looking through a culturally competent lens may also involve taking steps to promote an atmosphere of inclusion in your organization. Examples provided by Ohio Mental Health and Addiction Services (2019) include:

- Celebrate culturally significant events, milestones, and/or birthdays during lunch-time or at retreats.
- Recognize holidays like Yom Kippur (Judaism) or Ramadan (Islam) the way that traditional holidays like Christmas or Thanksgiving are.
- Develop a calendar of inclusive religious and cultural events.
- Include diverse people in institutional problem solving and decision-making.

To become a culturally competent healthcare provider, you must first understand yourself fully. Begin with examining yourself and your biases. Understanding our own perspectives is critical to uncovering potential negative bias (negative bias means that we can only remember unpleasant incidents). Bias can be extremely powerful when it operates below our consciousness or awareness. This is referred to as implicit bias, which is when people consciously reject stereotypes and support anti-discrimination efforts but also hold negative associations in their mind unconsciously. Implicit bias does not mean that they are hiding their perspective; rather, they are literally unaware that it exists. For example, anti-immigrant bias is the belief that a person is inferior because he or she immigrated to the United States from another country. Someone with an anti-immigrant bias might think, "I am accepting and supportive of immigrants" but still support policies that marginalize them. Another example is religious bias, the belief that people who belong to particular religious groups are inferior to members of other religious groups. Persons with a religious bias might unconsciously think that Christians are dominant and all other religions are subordinate. Our beliefs are often different from those we encounter every day, so we need to consider what these differences might be and how they could impact our interactions with others.

We must seek to uncover any implicit biases that we hold, as we can unknowingly convey them through our actions. Once we do this, it is important to look beyond ourselves and expand to new experiences, interactions, and conversations. This results in new dialogs of acceptance with our patients.

Applying Cultural Competence to Intersectional Identities and Needs

Intersectionality is defined as a "complex, cumulative way in which the effects of multiple forms of discrimination (such as racism, sexism, and classism) combine, overlap, or intersect especially in the experiences of marginalized individuals or groups" (Merriam-Webster, 2019). It is a theory that Kimberlé Williams Crenshaw developed in 1989 to explore the oppression and discrimination of women of color within society (Crenshaw, 1994). Crenshaw wrote that traditional feminist ideas and antiracist policies exclude African American women because they face overlapping discrimination: "Because the intersectional experience is greater than the sum of racism and sexism, any analysis that does not take *intersectionality* into account cannot sufficiently address the particular manner in which Black women are subordinated" (Crenshaw, 1994). Today the theory has expanded to include many more aspects of social identity and stratification, such as class, sexual orientation, age, religion, creed, and disability. It's vital to remember that cultural identity or affiliation with a particular group does not necessarily mean that an individual believes, observes, or practices every norm of that culture. For example, some Mexicans see themselves as "Latino," others as "Hispanic" or "Chicano." Your patients and coworkers bring many intersectional layers of culture with them, many of which are invisible. The theory of intersectionality does not mean that a certain combination of identities will always result in the same experiences; rather, it provides a way of understanding experiences through the lens of integrated identities.

Gender, income, and racial/ethnic identities intersect in working with low-income women of color. These multiple identities of social belonging can involve intersections and can vary across cultures. Assessing the barriers and facilitators related to racial or ethnic identity, income level, or the combination of the two is important for determining the best course of care for a patient. Intersections also interact with one another, influencing patients' experiences, possibilities, and challenges as well as providers' resources and capacity to provide cancer care support. For example, one's experiences are not separately determined by being a woman, an African American, and a low-income person. Rather, all of these qualities may exist in the same person, and the interaction between them determines the person's experiences. An African American woman who has a higher income may have a very different experience than a low-income African American woman, or even a low-income African American man. As a result, the way we approach a woman's problem or challenge must take into account the woman's availability of resources. These intersectional layers have important impacts on health access and outcomes.

Concepts of Difference in Health

We have all heard synonyms for the word "differences." But when we consider differences in health and why some groups have better outcomes than others, there is a trend away from "differences" and toward "equity" and "fairness." In this section, we will discuss three concepts of difference: health equity, health disparities, and social determinants of health. These concepts are important terms used to look at health and why some groups have better outcomes than others. Each term is slightly different, and the concepts should be distinguished when comparing one group to another. These terms are also related to social justice and improving the health of low-income women of color—and indeed all Americans. There are also often multiple, valid methods for assessing differences in health between populations.

Health Equity

The pursuit of health equity must remain at the forefront of our efforts. Health equity means that resources are fairly distributed among all segments of society and that everyone has an opportunity to be as healthy as possible, regardless of social or economic standing. This requires removing barriers, challenges, and obstacles to health such as discrimination and its consequences, such as powerlessness and lack of access to good jobs that offer fair pay, quality healthcare insurance coverage, and safe environments (Braveman et al., 2017). In contrast, health inequity means that health resources (like health insurance, education, flu vaccines, fresh food, and clean air) are distributed or allocated unfairly between diverse groups. Health equity is a desirable goal or standard that attempts to improve the health of those who have experienced social or economic disadvantage.

Health Disparities

Health disparities are preventable differences in the burden of disease or in opportunities to achieve optimal health experienced by socially disadvantaged women of color, women in poverty, and other disadvantaged groups and communities (National Academies of Sciences, Engineering, and Medicine, 2017). If a health outcome is seen to a greater or lesser extent between populations, there is a disparity. Disparities occur across many dimensions, including race/ethnicity, socioeconomic status, age, community, gender, insurance, and so forth. And as the U.S. population becomes increasingly diverse, health disparities will become even more prevalent if they are not adequately addressed. Here are a few examples of some common disparities seen within some groups as compared to others:

- Adults with disabilities are more likely to be obese, smoke, have high blood pressure, and be inactive than adults without disabilities. They are also three times more likely to have heart disease, stroke, diabetes, or cancer (Carroll et al., 2014; Courtney-Long et al., 2014; Stevens et al., 2014; Weil et al., 2002).
- African American infants are significantly more likely than non-Hispanic White and Hispanic infants to be born preterm and/or at a low birth weight, the two

leading causes of mortality among African American infants (Centers for Disease Control and Prevention, 2019).

- Less educated, low-income, and minority populations are less likely to have health insurance coverage, impairing their ability to access and afford care (National Research Council, 2004; Sohn, 2017).

So why do diversity and changing demographics matter in your role as a healthcare provider? This is important because as the United States diversifies, we might not understand certain populations and thus not be able to effectively assist these groups. According to 2018 population estimates recently released by the U.S. Census Bureau, the nation as a whole not only continues to grow older (with the median age increasing to 38.2 years in 2018, up from 37.2 years in 2010) (U.S. Census Bureau, 2019) but is also changing by race and ethnicity. Below are examples of changes in race and ethnicity compositions from the U.S. Census Bureau population estimates:

- Of the 50 states and the District of Columbia, 20 had a White population of 5 million or more, 21 were between 1.0 million and 4.9 million, nine were between 500,000 and 999,999, and one, the District of Columbia, had a population between 100,000 and 499,999.
- In 2018, 18 states had an African American population of 1 million or more.
- California was the only state to have an Asian population larger than 5 million (6,890,703 in 2018). New York (1,922,974) and Texas (1,688,966) were the only two states that had a population between 1 million and 4.9 million.
- The American Indian and Alaska Native population was over 1 million in only one state, California (1,089,694 in 2018).
- In 2018, 36 states and the District of Columbia had a Native Hawaiian and Other Pacific Islander population that was less than 20,000. The two states with the largest Native Hawaiian and Other Pacific Islander populations in 2018 were Hawaii (382,261) and California (363,437).
- In 2018, the Hispanic population was between 100,000 and 499,999 in 20 states. Among the states and the District of Columbia, 10 states had a Hispanic population of 1 million or more. California (15,540,142), Texas (11,368,849), and Florida (5,562,417) were the only states that had Hispanic populations of 5 million or more.

With regard to women specifically, 2017 statistics show that they are 38% more likely than men to live in poverty (National Women's Law Center, 2016). And when broken down by race, additional poverty disparities appear (National Women's Law Center, 2017): 21% of African American women, 20% of Native women, 18% of Latina women, 11% of Asian women, and 9% of White, non-Hispanic women live in poverty.

As the population becomes more diverse, it is a business and social justice imperative for healthcare providers to recognize the need to deliver culturally competent care and services to improve health outcomes, lower the total cost of care, and improve patient satisfaction (Cigna Corporation, 2016). Not only race but also class, gender, and culture can lead to disparities within our healthcare systems. There are many issues that contribute to disparities in health, such as variations in access to care and quality of care; language barriers and health literacy; and issues of trust or mistrust in the healthcare system and medical bias toward specific groups. In addition, social determinants of health, such as socioeconomic status and educational attainment, can contribute to health disparities.

There are opportunities to address health disparities through cultural competency. Health disparities represent more than a medical and scientific issue; they are also a social justice issue and a moral commitment to understanding and addressing many of the racial, economic, age, and gender inequities and injustices faced by low-income women of color throughout the cancer care spectrum.

Social Determinants of Health

Social determinants of health are the environmental conditions in which people are born, live, learn, work, play, worship, and age that affect a wide range of health, functioning, and quality-of-life outcomes and risks (Healthy People 2030, 2021). Social determinants include physical characteristics that are observable (such as age, race, sexual orientation or identity, and gender) as well as circumstances shaped by a wider set of influences and systems put in place to deal with illness (like employment opportunities, insurance, income, housing, transportation, access to fresh fruits/vegetables, etc.). Negative social determinants of health include poverty, poor access to education, unhealthy housing, and exposure to general disadvantage. The result of such adverse factors can be an increased risk of cancer and other diseases (Rodriguez, 2017). Addressing the social determinants of health has the potential to improve healthcare and the overall health of everyone.

National Standards for Culturally and Linguistically Appropriate Services

Culturally and linguistically appropriate services (CLAS) is one strategy to improve the quality of services provided to all individuals, which will ultimately help reduce health disparities and achieve health equity (U.S. Department of Health and Human Services, 2019). The CLAS standards include a set of 15 action steps that healthcare organizations can use to advance health equity and help eliminate health disparities. The action steps are categorized into three overarching themes: (1) Governance, Leadership, and Workforce; (2) Communication and Language Assistance; and (3) Engagement, Continuous Improvement, and Accountability (U.S. Department of Health and Human Services, 2019). The principal standard is to provide effective, equitable, understandable, and respectful quality care and services that are responsive to diverse cultural health beliefs and practices, preferred languages, health literacy, and other communication needs (U.S. Department of Health and Human Services, 2019). By tailoring their interventions to an individual's culture and language preference, healthcare providers can effect change and improve health care outcomes among diverse populations.

Other Important Cultural Competency Concepts

Understanding women whose cultural background is not the same as yours is critical to cultural competency. In this section, we will present several concepts important to consider when practicing as a culturally competent healthcare provider: cultural humility, cultural sensitivity, and cultural awareness.

Cultural Humility

Cultural humility is different from the other two culturally based concepts because it focuses on self-humility, rather than achieving knowledge or awareness of the patient. Cultural humility is the ability to maintain an interpersonal position that is sensitive and humble to the aspects of cultural identity most important to the patient. For example, if religion and spirituality are critical to your patient, it would be important for you to focus on your cultural humility with regard to this aspect of her beliefs and practices in health care. Below is a list of some of the common religious denominations in the United States, with their corresponding beliefs and health practices. For healthcare providers, of course, cultural competence goes far beyond this list; improving our communication with and understanding of patients from different backgrounds and cultures represents a continuous and lifelong endeavor (Ehman, 2012; Rumun, 2014).

- **Armenian:** Beliefs reflect no conflict between modern medicine and religion. Traditionally, baptism involves immersion eight days after birth. Confirmation is done immediately after baptism. On the fortieth day after birth, the parents bring the child to church. Armenians advocate taking communion and the laying on of hands.
- **Baha'i:** Beliefs reflect no conflict between modern medicine and religion. The sick are specifically instructed in Baha'i scriptures to seek the advice of competent doctors. Spiritual health is thought to be conducive to physical health. Prayer is an adjunct to healing by physical and chemical means and is considered legitimate or even indispensable. They do not adhere to baptism practices. Members advise prayer and, if medically permissible, fasting.
- **Baptist:** Organ transplants are generally approved when they do not seriously endanger the donor and when they offer real medical hope for the recipient. Baptists do not attribute any physically healing powers to baptism or communion. These rights are understood by Baptists as "ordinances" rather than "sacraments" because the latter term suggests that the elements of these rites are "means of grace" and that they somehow transfer "power" from God to the recipient. Some Baptists believe in and practice healing by the laying on of hands.
- **Black Muslim:** General adherence to Muslim tenets is overlain in many instances by antagonism to Caucasians, especially Christians and Jews. They do not indulge in activities (such as sleeping) more than is necessary to health and always maintain personal habits of cleanliness. They do not adhere to baptism practices. Faith healing is not acceptable among Black Muslims.
- **Buddhist Churches of America:** They are in harmony with modern science. They believe there is no divine punishment. This is a religion of supreme optimism, as it teaches a way to overcome fears, anxieties, and apprehension. Rites such as infant presentation, affirmation, confirmation, and ordination are performed after the child has become mature enough. A Buddhist priest should be notified for counseling, but it should be at the patient's or family's request.
- **Church of Jesus Christ of Latter-day Saints:** Members who are hospitalized need the assurance of God and the fellowship of fellow saints. Religious sacraments (like communion, laying on of hands, anointing with oil, and counseling by a minister) are not practiced by the church. Organ transplants are not a religious problem.

- **Islam (Muslim):** They often have a fatalistic view that can militate against ready compliance with therapy. The Five Pillars of Islam are five practices regarded by all sects as essential to the Muslim faith: (1) Shahadah: sincerely reciting the Muslim profession of faith; (2) Salat: performing ritual prayers in the proper way five times each day; (3) Zakat: paying an alms (or charity) tax to benefit the poor and the needy; (4) Sawm: fasting during the month of Ramadan; and (5) Hajj: pilgrimage to Mecca. Other notable Islamic practices include the mystical rituals of Sufism and various distinctive Shi'ite practices. Faith healing is for the patient's morale only; conservative members reject medical therapy.
- **Jehovah's Witnesses:** They believe the Bible is the word of God. They practice giving out information and statements found in the Bible to the public. Generally, they will not accept blood transfusions; a court order may be required for an emergency transfusion.
- **Judaism:** Believe in organ transplantation only if it is to save the life of a patient or improve his or her health, but most believe the sanctity of the human body covers each of its members and organs. Thus, any part of the body that is separated from the corpus also requires burial. Whenever possible, the family and rabbi should be present when a patient seems ready to pass away. There is a special confession called Vidui that is recited at that time.
- **Lutheran:** Most members believe that transplanting organs from a deceased to a living person is a genuine medical advance. The Lutheran Church recognizes baptism and the Lord's Supper as sacraments. If the prognosis is poor, the patient may request anointment and blessing.
- **Methodist, United:** Baptism for children or adults. Two sacraments are recognized: baptism and Holy Communion. Communication may be requested prior to surgery or a similar crisis.
- **Native Americans:** Religious beliefs, magic, folklore, disease treatment, and herbal medicine differ from tribe to tribe. Some follow modern Christian religions and practices, whereas others continue with traditional beliefs. Protection against disease is sought by the help of superhuman powers.
- **Pentecostal (Assembly of God, Foursquare Church):** They believe in water baptism by immersion after age of accountability. Some insist illness is a divine punishment, but most consider illness an intrusion of Satan. Deliverance from sin and sickness is provided for by atonement. There are no prohibitions on blood transfusions or medical care. Members believe in the possibility of divine healing through prayer. Anointing with oil may be practiced with laying on of hands.
- **Roman Catholic:** Infant baptism is mandatory and is especially urgent if the baby's prognosis is poor. Baptism is demanded if an aborted fetus may not be clinically dead. Roman Catholics usually go to Mass on Sundays and on holidays such as Christmas and Easter. The patient or family may desire that an amputated limb be buried in consecrated ground; there is no mandate for this, although it may be required by a given diocese.
- **Russian Orthodox:** It is important not to shave male patients except in preparation for surgery. Baptism is done by a priest only. The wearing of a cross necklace is important. and it should be replaced immediately when a patient returns from surgery.

We don't need to be cultural information experts, but we do need to show humility with our patients' religious and cultural beliefs and practices. It is important to view each interaction as a learning opportunity to improve our cultural competency.

Cultural Sensitivity

Cultural sensitivity involves being aware that cultural differences and similarities exist and affect our values, learning, and behavior. Being culturally sensitive means trying to be aware of and to respect different beliefs and behaviors and to accommodate these where possible. Beyond that, we must celebrate and affirm our differences, creating an inclusive environment where patients and other providers feel comfortable and confident coming into the healthcare institution. An example might be asking your patient, "How would you like to be addressed?" and making a note in the chart of her preference. Patient forms could include a range of partnership statuses: single, married, domestic partnership, divorced, or widowed.

Cultural Awareness

Cultural awareness represents the foundation of cultural competency and involves developing a sensitivity to and understanding of another ethnic group (Asian Health Support Services, 2010). It captures both cultural humility and cultural sensitivity but goes beyond them. Cultural awareness involves the ability to stand back from ourselves and become aware of our own cultural values, beliefs, and perceptions. If you recognize your own values and biases, as well as the values and biases of your patients, and be consciously aware of your reaction and the reaction of your patients, then you can monitor your attitudes and behaviors so you can interact appropriately and have more satisfying health outcomes (Asian Health Support Services, 2010). For example, in working with older African American women, it is important for you to acknowledge any racism and/or sexism in the environment. It is also important to recognize that mistrust, aggravated by the lack of diversity within the healthcare institution, can reduce the likelihood that an individual will proactively seek care and/or adhere to healthcare recommendations.

Providers must understand their own values and beliefs and not allow them to affect their practice. In a patient–provider relationship, the provider is responsible for promoting trust by ensuring there is no power differential and by following ethical codes of practice and boundaries.

While we have reviewed important cultural competency concepts and now have a better understanding, remaining culturally competent is an ongoing process. We can always learn more and do better. Table 1.1 lists additional concepts and definitions relevant to cultural competence in real-world settings. While no single pocket guide, course, or training can make any one healthcare provider culturally competent, we can learn valuable concepts and tools and develop strategies in our healthcare settings with low-income women of color. The most important thing to remember is that you are responsible for your own "cultural health." This also means addressing cultural competency within the institutions we serve. Just as we support our patients, we should support our fellow healthcare providers across the board. Providers need to be diverse to understand and meet the needs of the women and populations we serve. This might mean tapping into our coworkers' journeys from time to time and viewing our challenges through their unique lenses. Cultural competency at the individual, interpersonal, and institutional level is the foundation of health communication.

Table 1.1 Concepts of Cultural Competency

Cultural Competency Concept	Definition
Bias	A prejudice in favor of or against one thing, person, or group compared with another, usually in a way considered to be unfair. It is a bend, a leaning, a strong inclination of the mind or a preconceived opinion about something or someone. *Implicit bias* refers to the attitudes or stereotypes that affect our understanding, actions, and decisions in an <u>unconscious</u> manner. On the other hand, *explicit bias* refers to the attitudes and beliefs we have about a person or group on a <u>conscious</u> level.
Bigotry	Extreme negative attitudes leading to hatred of a group and persons regarded as members of the group.
Culture	Customs, norms, beliefs, values, practices, and social institutions, including religious and spiritual traditions.
Cultural blindness	Providers deny any differences between groups and assume that practices used with the majority population, generally Whites, may work equally as well with minority non-Whites.
Cultural competence	A continuous learning process that builds knowledge, awareness, skills, and capacity to identify, understand, and respect the unique beliefs, values, customs, language, abilities, and traditions of all, in order to develop policies to promote effective programs and services.
Discrimination	The act of treating a person, issue, or behavior unjustly or unequally as a result of prejudices; a showing of partiality or prejudice in treatment; specific actions or policies directed against the welfare of minority groups. Occurs when people are treated differently based on stereotypical beliefs combined with prejudicial attitudes and emotions, like fear and hostility.
Diversity	The state of being unique and varied.
Ethnicity	A social construct that divides people into social groups based on characteristics, like language, a common history, and national origin. Every race has a variety of ethnic groups.
Fatalism	The belief that all events are predetermined and therefore inevitable and that individuals cannot do much to alter their fate.
Health disparities	Differences in health status between segments of the population due to greater social and/or economic barriers to health.
Institutional racism	A form of racism expressed in the practice of social and political institutions. It is reflected in disparities regarding wealth, income, criminal justice, employment, housing, healthcare, political power and education, among other factors.
Intersectionality	A complex, cumulative way in which the effects of multiple forms of discrimination (such as racism, sexism, and classism) combine, overlap, or intersect, especially in the experiences of marginalized individuals or groups.
	The roots of poverty, classism, and racism that are linked to the socio-political and socio-historical factors that marginalize and oppress. Examples include: • Ableism: the belief that a disabled person is inferior to someone who does not have a disability. • Ageism: the belief that young people are superior to elderly people. • Classism: treating a person as inferior based on social class (middle and upper classes are dominant; poor and working classes are subordinate).

(continued)

Table 1.1 Continued

Cultural Competency Concept	Definition
"-Isms"	• Homophobia: prejudice and discrimination against someone because of his or her perceived or actual sexual orientation. • Linguicism: the belief that a person is inferior based on the language he or she speaks (English speakers are dominant; all other languages are subordinate). • Racism: the belief that one person is inferior to another based on his or her skin color (White people belong to the dominant group; people of color make up the subordinate group). • Sexism: the belief that a person is inferior based on his or her sex (men are dominant; women and transgender people are subordinate).
LGBTQIA	Acronym or lesbian, gay, bisexual, transgender, queer or questioning, intersex, and asexual or allied.
Marginalization	Treatment of a person or group as insignificant or pushing people to the edge of society by not allowing them a place within it.
Microaggression	Everyday verbal, nonverbal, and environmental slights, snubs, or insults, whether intentional or unintentional, that communicate hostile, derogatory, or negative messages to target persons based solely upon their marginalized group membership.
Oppression	When members of a dominant group possess privilege that gives them power not afforded to subordinate groups.
Prejudice	A negative attitude toward a group or persons perceived to be members of that group; being predisposed to behave negatively toward members of a group. Can be based on gender, ethnicity, race, socioeconomic status.
Race	Category to which others assign individuals on the basis of physical characteristics such as skin color or hair type.
Stereotype	Usually a negative trait or belief about a particular group ascribed to most members of that group.
White privilege	The benefits of access to resources and social rewards, and the power to shape the norms and values of society, that White individuals receive by virtue of their position in society.

References

Asian Health Support Services. (2010). *Cultural and cultural competency workbook*. Waitemata District Health Board.

Braveman, P., Arkin, E., Orleans, T., Proctor, D., & Plough, A., (2017). What is health equity? Robert Wood Johnson Foundation. https://www.rwjf.org/en/library/research/2017/05/what-is-health-equity-.html

Carroll, D., Courtney-Long, E., Stevens, A., Sloan, M., Lullo, C., Visser, S., Fox, M., Armour, B., Campbell, V., Brown, D., & Dorn, J. M., & Centers for Disease Control and Prevention (CDC) (2014). Vital signs: disability and physical activity—United States, 2009–2012. *MMWR. Morbidity and Mortality Weekly Report, 63*(18), 407–413.

Centers for Disease Control and Prevention. (2019). Preterm health. https://www.cdc.gov/reproductivehealth/maternalinfanthealth/pretermbirth.htm

Cigna Corporation. (2016). Cultural competency in health care. https://www.cigna.com/assets/docs/about-cigna/thn-white-papers/cultural-competency-in-health-care-final.pdf

Courtney-Long, E., Stevens, A., Caraballo, R., Ramon, I., & Armour, B. S. (2014). Disparities in current cigarette smoking prevalence by type of disability, 2009–2011. *Public Health Reports, 129*(3), 252–60.

Crenshaw, K. (1994). Intersectionality [video]. TED Conferences. https://elon.libguides.com/antiracism/intersectionality

Cross, T. L., Bazron, B. J., Dennis, K. W., & Isaacs, M. R. (1989). *Towards a culturally competent system of care.* Washington, DC: Georgetown University Child Development Center.

Ehman, J. (2012). *Religious diversity: Practical points for health care providers.* Department of Pastoral Care, Hospital of the University of Pennsylvania & Penn Presbyterian Medical Center, Philadelphia, PA.

Healthy People 2030. (2021). U.S. Department of Health and Human Services, Office of Disease Prevention and Health Promotion. https://health.gov/healthypeople/objectives-and-data/social-determinants-health

Iwamoto, D. K., & Liu, W. M. (2010). The impact of racial identity, ethnic identity, Asian values and race-related stress on Asian Americans and Asian international college students' psychological well-being. *Journal of Counseling Psychology, 57*(1), 79–91. doi:10.1037/a0017393

Lum, D. (2011). *Culturally competent practice: A framework for understanding diverse groups and justice issues,* 4th ed. Brooks/Cole.

Merriam-Webster. (2019). Intersectionality. In *Merriam-Webster's collegiate dictionary.* https://www.merriam-webster.com/dictionary/intersectionality

National Academies of Sciences, Engineering, and Medicine. (2017). The root causes of health inequity. In *Communities in action: Pathways to health equity.* National Academies Press, 99–184. doi:10.17226/24624

National Research Council Panel on Race, Ethnicity, and Health in Later Life; Bulatao, R. A., & Anderson, N. B. (Eds.) (2004). *Understanding Racial and Ethnic Differences in Health in Late Life: A Research Agenda.* National Academies Press, 10, Health Care. https://www.ncbi.nlm.nih.gov/books/NBK24693/

National Women's Law Center. (2017). NWLC resources on poverty, income, and health insurance in 2016. https://nwlc.org/resources/nwlc-resources-on-poverty-income-and-health-insurance-in-2016/

Ohio Mental Health and Addiction Services. (2016). Fairfield County Alcohol, Drug Addiction, and Mental Health (ADAMH) Board Community Plan. https://mha.ohio.gov/Portals/0/assets/SchoolsAndCommunities/CommunityAndHousing/Community-Planning/2014/Fairfield%202014%20Community%20Plan.pdf?ver=2018-12-17-112647-840

Ohio Mental Health and Addiction Services. (2019). *Cultural competence in mental health and addiction recovery.* Ohio eBased Academy.

Rodriguez, A. (2017). Addressing social determinant factors that negatively impact an individual's health. AJMC Managed Markets and Network. https://www.ajmc.com/newsroom/social-determinant-factors-can-negatively-impact-an-individuals-health

Rumun, A. J. (2014). Influence of religious beliefs on healthcare practice. *International Journal of Education and Research, 2,* 37–48.

Sohn, H. (2017). Racial and ethnic disparities in health insurance coverage: Dynamics of gaining and losing coverage over the life-course. *Population Research and Policy Review, 36*(2), 181–201. doi:10.1007/s11113-016-9416-y

Stevens, A., Courtney-Long, E., Gillespie, C., & Armour, B. S. (2014). Hypertension among US adults by disability status and type, National Health and Nutrition Examination Survey, 2001–2010. *Preventing Chronic Disease, 11,* E139.

U.S. Census Bureau. (2019). Population estimates show aging across race groups differs. https://www.census.gov/newsroom/press-releases/2019/estimates-characteristics.html

U.S. Department of Health and Human Services. (2019). Think Cultural Health: National culturally and linguistically appropriate services standards. https://www.thinkculturalhealth.hhs.gov/clas/standards

Villa, M. L., Cuellar, J., Gamel, N., & Yeo, G. (1993). *Aging and health: Hispanic American elders* (2nd edition). SGEC Working Paper Series, Number 5, Ethnogeriatric Reviews, Stanford Geriatric Education Center.

Weil, E., Wachterman, M., McCarthy, E. P., Davis, R. B., O'Day, B., Iezzoni, L. I., & Wee, C. C. (2002). Obesity among adults with disabling conditions. *Journal of the American Medical Association, 288*, 1265–1268.

Chapter 1 Takeaways

- The goal of the healthcare provider should be to communicate in a way that educates the patient, while also uplifting her sense of self-efficacy and motivating her to take control of her health.
- To improve follow-up rates among low-income women of color, providers must be aware of adherence facilitators (e.g., spirituality, social support) as well as barriers (e.g., psychosocial needs, stressors), particularly given that many of these barriers exist at the system level and providers are often responsible for initial cancer screenings.
- Cultural competency represents the foundation of health communication. Providers must be culturally competent so they can help women solve problems, make informed decisions, feel empowered, and place trust in their healthcare providers and the healthcare system.

2
Intervention and Strategies Across the Cancer Continuum

> Patient navigator: "What I hear from women in their position is, 'Okay, so now I've found something wrong. I have no money. I have no resources. How am I going to now care for my kids, care for my aging parents, care for myself; what is that going to look like, how am I going to access this care when I don't have a pot to throw out the window?'"
>
> Wells et al., 2019, p. 57

Chapter 2 provides an overview and examples of how various communication strategies and interventions can be used to support and improve screening and treatment adherence among low-income women of color. The impact of unique values, beliefs, and cultural practices on health education and behavior is discussed, and recommendations for application are made in cancer and communication across the cancer continuum.

Module 2.1: Patient Navigation

This module introduces evidence-based interventions and strategies across the cancer continuum. We discuss the importance of patient navigation for women of color and the ingredients and skills needed to implement a patient navigation program. We have found that when attempting to encourage nonadherent or hard-to-reach women to initiate and maintain cancer screening, it is most important to focus on four areas: problem solving, information, motivation, and behaviors. The relevance of problem solving for addressing adherence barriers related to preventing cancer or treating cancer is embedded in coping with stressful circumstances. Information is a critical component and can include relevant research data, health promotion information, preventive or risk details about cancer or screening or treatment behavior, and information on positive outcomes from screening or treatment initiation and maintenance. Using motivational strategies has been proven to enhance adherence efforts. Behavioral skills are also critical determinants of health that influence whether well-informed and well-motivated individuals are capable of carrying out a health behavior effectively.

Cancer Navigation. Anjanette A. Wells, Vetta L. Sanders Thompson, Will Ross, Carol Camp Yeakey, and Sheri R. Notaro, Oxford University Press. © Oxford University Press 2022. DOI: 10.1093/med/9780190672867.003.0003

What Is Patient Navigation?

Patient navigation is a central tool of the expanded chronic care model (CCM), as it helps patients to move through the process of screening, diagnosis, treatment, and recovery in a personalized fashion, with the assistance of knowledgeable guides. Patient navigation was developed by Harold Freeman, MD, while working in Harlem, New York, with a population that consisted of predominately low-income African American women. Patient navigation is a widely accepted evidence-based intervention and was a key feature of the Patient Protection and Affordable Care Act (ACA) (2010) (Freeman, 2006; Howard et al., 2007). It was designed to improve cancer disparities by reducing screening adherence barriers and increasing screening rates through flexible problem-solving techniques, particularly at diagnostic follow-up and in the treatment setting among lower socioeconomic status and racial/ethnic minority populations. Such barriers can be particularly problematic when trying to use evidence-based interventions to improve health for medically underserved populations and residents in under-resourced areas because so few interventions are tested in these situations. By assessing barriers and building interventions based on those barriers, patient navigation's effectiveness can be seen in the use of randomized trials testing with minority populations (Percac-Lima et al., 2008; Ravenell et al., 2013). Based on a social support theoretical underpinning, navigation services can be provided by a lay peer navigator or a community health worker (Hunt et al., 2017; Lobb & Colditz, 2013). With roots in combining community and culturally sensitive care coordination with aspects of disease management, navigation has been shown to improve adherence by assessing and alleviating personal and systems-level barriers.

Navigation can support women throughout the cancer continuum, from screening through diagnosis, treatment, survivorship, and end-of-life care (Hopkins & Mumber, 2009). Navigation stages include:

1. Primary preventive screening outreach: adoption of healthy lifestyles and disease prevention
2. Diagnosis: removal of barriers to accessing screening
3. Treatment: education, support, and coordination of multidisciplinary care and providing resources and referrals
4. Survivorship: wellness, stress management, education, long-term care plans, and support groups (Hopkins & Mumber, 2009).

Our training experience with Dr. Freeman at the Harold P. Freeman Patient Navigation Institute in January 2012 and our practice experience have reinforced critical elements of the navigation process. According to the Institute's training, patient navigation involves the following core principles (Freeman & Rodriguez, 2011):

1. Navigation is a patient-centric healthcare service delivery model.
2. Patient navigation serves to virtually integrate a fragmented healthcare system for the individual patient.
3. The core function of patient navigation is the elimination of barriers to timely care across all segments of the healthcare continuum.
4. Patient navigation should be defined with a clear scope of practice that distinguishes the role and responsibilities of the navigator from that of other providers.

5. Delivery of patient navigation services should be cost-effective and commensurate with the training and skills necessary to guide an individual through a particular phase of the care continuum.
6. The person doing the navigating should be determined by the level of skills required at a given phase of navigation.
7. In a given system of care, there is the need to define the point at which navigation ends.
8. There is a need to navigate patients across disconnected systems of care, such as primary-care sites and tertiary-care sites.
9. Patient navigation systems require coordination.

Often patient navigation process never ends, as it includes the phases of prevention, early detection, diagnosis, treatment, the posttreatment period, and survivorship. Survivorship is often the least developed phase of the continuum.

One primary goal of navigation is to help reduce cancer disparities by increasing cancer screening rates (Paskett et al., 2011; Vargas et al., 2008; Yosha, 2011), particularly among underserved, poor, and minority populations (Ferrante, 2007). Patient navigation is an evidence-based intervention approach (Hendren et al., 2010) shown to improve adherence by assessing and alleviating personal (e.g., financial strain, complex domestic/interpersonal relationships, lack of access to transportation, poor health, lack of social support) and systems-level barriers to care (e.g., multiple clinic appointments, eligibility requirements, clinical follow-up for abnormal results). Patient navigators assist individuals in completing recommended cancer screening, additional testing, and treatment (Vargas et al., 2008; Yosha, 2011). They also help individuals to efficiently navigate the intricacies of the healthcare system, and they work across the continuum of care (Calhoun et al., 2010; Parker et al., 2010; Vargas et al., 2008) by facilitating relationships with health clinics, determining eligibility for services, ensuring accessibility for participants, and addressing individual concerns regarding screening.

Training for Patient Navigators

A primary objective of patient navigation is to reduce obstacles to preventive care and to improve the delivery of care (Pederson & Hack, 2010). This barrier-reduction approach (Calhoun et al., 2010; Parker et al., 2010) is typically conducted by trained patient navigators who (1) have a bachelor's or higher degree in the health, social, or behavioral sciences (e.g., health education, psychology, and other related disciplines); (2) have experience working with diverse populations and strong communication skills (Shelton et al., 2011); and (3) are knowledgeable about the resources in their community. Often navigators are able to relate to the individuals they serve because they come from similar cultural backgrounds (Darnell, 2007; Wells et al., 2011).

Based on our experience, initial training sessions for patient navigators should use multiple learning modalities, including traditional lectures, interactive formats, and role plays with case scenarios (Shelton et al., 2011). The training should provide an overview of evidence-based cancer control, cultural competency, barriers to care, problem-solving techniques, basic counseling concepts and approaches, resource mapping (McKenney et al., 2018; Wells et al., 2008), and documentation. During this time, navigators should receive clinical oversight from supervisors. Over the first several months of a patient navigation program or service, patient navigators should receive weekly or biweekly individual and group supervision to review documentation and feedback. It is best if these sessions also include discussion of challenging cases, review of participant flow, identification of new resources, and problem solving related to process improvement (Vargas et al., 2008).

Starting the Patient Navigation Process

Patient navigators can start the process by phoning a woman to introduce themselves and their role, explain the navigation relationship, address the woman's current needs, and establish rapport. Immediately after completing this introductory call, the navigator can send the woman a letter or postcard containing the navigator's name, picture, and contact information. This correspondence can also include a mission statement, stated in lay language, which helps to guide the relationship (Figure 2.1). The patient navigator can subsequently contact the woman to make sure she received the letter or postcard and to answer any questions or follow up on any issues resulting from the initial conversation.

Navigators should make sure that patients are aware of the ways the many ways the navigator can assist them. The list in Figure 2.2 can be shared with patients in correspondence and in the initial introductory session.

Subsequent conversations can include discussion about ways to address questions and concerns related to behavioral action (e.g., scheduling an appointment for screening, arranging transportation for screening). Through regular sustained contact, the patient navigator should work collaboratively with the woman as a partner to empower her to prioritize her own health and self-care through a focus on problem solving, information, motivation, and behavioral skills.

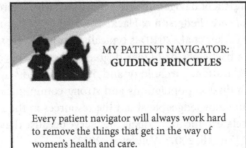

MY PATIENT NAVIGATOR:
GUIDING PRINCIPLES

Every patient navigator will always work hard to remove the things that get in the way of women's health and care.

Every patient navigator will support and "stand up for" women who experience many different and important needs.

Figure 2.1 Guiding principles

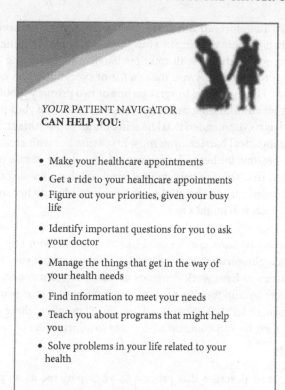

YOUR PATIENT NAVIGATOR
CAN HELP YOU:

- Make your healthcare appointments
- Get a ride to your healthcare appointments
- Figure out your priorities, given your busy life
- Identify important questions for you to ask your doctor
- Manage the things that get in the way of your health needs
- Find information to meet your needs
- Teach you about programs that might help you
- Solve problems in your life related to your health

Figure 2.2 Patient navigator information sheet

Problem Solving

An important feature of patient navigation is the use of problem solving (Wells et al., 2015). The relevance of problem solving for addressing adherence barriers related to preventing cancer or treating cancer is embedded in coping with stressful circumstances. Problem-solving skills are important to moderating the relationship between the woman's life stressors and the need to adhere to her health care. Many patient navigation programs incorporate in this process the sociocultural nuances of women they serve (Ell et al., 2008; Percac-Lima et al., 2009). This is why systematic problem-solving techniques should be customized to women of color, particularly when socio-environmental stressors are a significant factor.

Problem solving teaches patients to address current life problems and stressors (e.g., deaths, separation or divorce, health problems in significant others, caregiving, economic problems, employment or unemployment issues) by identifying smaller elements of larger problems and developing specific steps toward solving these problems. The evidence-based intervention called Problem Solving Treatment (PST) (Nezu et al., 1994) is a cognitive-behavioral treatment that has been found effective in improving psychosocial coping among minorities with daily life stressors and comorbidities. PST is a highly structured process that generally includes six to eight sessions, which is often not feasible in the time-limited settings that we work in with this population (University of

Washington, 2019). Therefore, an abbreviated version is likely more congruent with the needs of healthcare providers working in a busy clinic or hospital setting.

Problem solving with patients with multiple barriers is like spring cleaning. When you get ready for spring cleaning, you make a list of everything you need to do to get ready for the season. First, you have to agree on one or two primary problems to work on, often among multiple confounding barriers (Wells et al., 2017). If your patient's problem is that her doctor has recommended that she schedule an appointment, yet she has multiple practical and logistical barriers, you must first assist her with creating a list of barriers or a menu of reasons for her lack of screening. You might decide to add to that list your observed concerns. This is a very concrete and collaborative way to begin to assist your patient, particularly when she might not be able to identify her main concerns or problems. For example, you might say,

> I am your patient navigator, and I would like to help you with any problems you are currently struggling with that make it difficult for you to get your mammogram. Some women like you have work demands or transportation concerns that might make it difficult to go into the clinic to get a mammogram. I hear you have some of the same concerns, so let's talk about this. Can you tell me about these problems, one at a time? And then we can come up with a way to address one or two of the most important ones.

You may choose to describe this process to your patients as a "problem funnel" (Figure 2.3). This funnel is wide enough at the top to accept all of your patient's barriers but narrow enough at the bottom to accommodate one or two agreed-upon barriers that are feasible to work on. This drilling-down process of problem solving involves seeking out all available facts about the problem from the woman's perspective and using clear and objective language. In your conversation, it is important to separate facts from assumptions. Attempt to unpack the woman's complex problems into smaller components. Then, based on these smaller problems, work with her to identify realistic goals and a feasible plan. This brainstorming and troubleshooting should be a collaborative effort, with the end goal of screening or treatment recommendation adherence.

The reality is that not all of the problems your patients face can be fixed or addressed within the timeframe or with the resources that the two of you have, particularly when the impediments involve financial obstacles. Socioeconomic class may greatly affect problem solving, given the different levels of financial and other resources available to people confronting these problems (Heppner et al., 2004). So for an unscreened woman, barrier-reduction activities, combined with problem solving, might be needed first (and throughout) to address the daily stressors, practical issues, and circumstances faced among those living in poverty. Studies show that those who live in poverty consider meeting their basic human needs as more important than obtaining cancer prevention and screening (Kreuter, 2016). The idea is to guide women in selecting problems that have a manageable, timely solution that they can carry out in order to reach the goal of adherence. The basic premise of problem solving is that if patients learn to identify and resolve problems, they will gain an increased sense of self-efficacy, control, and confidence while becoming more active in obtaining rewards and satisfaction from their environment. Gradually, patients will take a more prominent role in problem solving, requiring less input and guidance from their patient navigator.

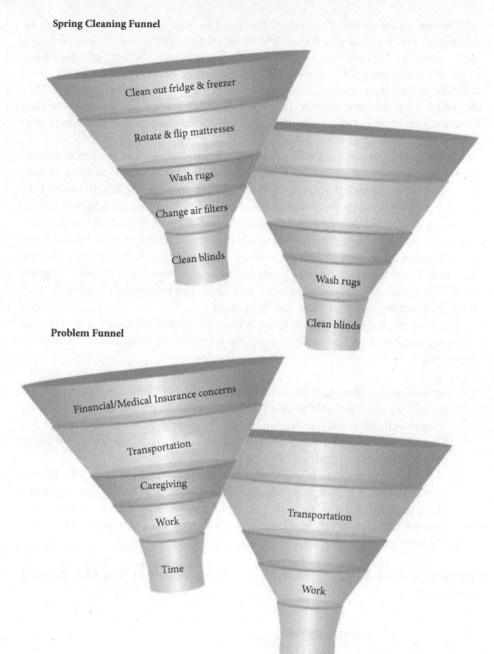

Spring Cleaning Funnel

Clean out fridge & freezer

Rotate & flip mattresses

Wash rugs

Change air filters

Clean blinds

Wash rugs

Clean blinds

Problem Funnel

Financial/Medical Insurance concerns

Transportation

Caregiving

Work

Time

Transportation

Work

Figure 2.3 Problem-solving funnel

Information

One part of solving problems involves obtaining accurate information such as relevant research data, health promotion information, preventive or risk details about cancer or screening or treatment behavior, and facts about positive outcomes from screening or treatment initiation and maintenance. In our prior research and practice experience with breast cancer survivors, we found that prior to women's diagnosis they were familiar with breast cancer as a disease and its seriousness, but they also perceived their susceptibility and risk to be low, particularly if a cancer history did not personally affect them or a family member (Wells et al., 2013). According to survivors, family members often did not talk about cancer, hid it, or considered it inappropriate for discussion. They described some common misperceptions that likely contributed to delay in screening behavior, like "there is radiation in the mammogram machine, which can cause breast cancer" (Wells et al., 2013).

It is critical for patient navigators to provide accurate information to overcome communication and informational barriers like these. Reinforcing this information with active one-on-one interactions and conversations can enhance the effectiveness of the educational portion of the intervention (Carrasquillo et al., 2018,). In addition, the information provided should be culturally tailored for this population (Diclemente, 2010; Kreuter et al., 2004; Skinner, 1994). There is evidence that offering tailored information that addresses the woman's specific screening and cancer risk status is more effective than simply providing standardized printed recommendations (Ell et al., 2008; Lopez & Castro, 2006). In addition, the information and advice that you provide needs to be reinforced as a part of the conversation with the patient.

Based on the findings of randomized studies of tailored educational cancer control interventions with low-income populations, materials should have three main components:

1. An educational message about cancer and the risks of delayed screening, written in lay language (possibly information obtained through the American Cancer Society or the National Institutes of Health/National Cancer Institute)
2. Clear information about local referrals and resources needed for women to obtain cancer screening or treatment
3. A short narrative example of a similar low-income woman of color who is overcoming a barrier (Champion & Scott, 1997; Russell et al., 2007). This might be a short personal story from an African American woman who appears to be between 40 and 70 years old and has received a mammogram screening even though she has a low income.

Information that is culturally tailored and language concordant is best (Percac-Lima et al., 2008).

Motivation

Even though is it an essential part of adherence and preventive health behavior, information alone is not enough, because well-informed individuals are not necessarily motivated to engage in favorable cancer behaviors (Fisher & Fisher, 2000) and tend to their health. For this reason, patient navigators should include motivational techniques in their work with women. Motivational strategies have proven to enhance adherence efforts (Pudkasam et al., 2018, 70; Tatum & Houston, 2017). For example, mammogram screening rates improved in an urban emergency department when women were offered a brief motivational interview, as well as traditional referral and a no-cost appointment the next day (Bernstein et al., 2000). Motivational techniques are relatively easy to integrate into current practice. In our experience, healthcare providers can be more intentional about the language they use to gently motivate patients.

Motivational interviewing (MI) is defined as

a collaborative, goal-oriented style of communication with particular attention to the language of change. It is designed to strengthen personal motivation for and commitment to a specific goal by eliciting and exploring the person's own reasons for change within an atmosphere of acceptance and compassion. (Miller & Rollnick, 2012, p. 29)

MI interventions have been used in a variety of illness and disease domains. Adherence to disease management involves unique behaviors and related challenges and barriers that are important to recognize. Table 2.1 lists studies that have used motivational techniques to improve adherence by addressing psychosocial barriers to specific illness and disease domains.

Based on the "stages of change" transtheoretical model, MI uses research to inform practice changes and emphasizes two specific active components: (1) a relational component focused on empathy and the interpersonal spirit of MI and (2) a technical component involving the differential evocation and reinforcement of "change talk" (Miller & Rolnick, 2012).

Table 2.1 Studies That Have Used Motivational Techniques to Improve Adherence

Illness/Disease Domain	Adherence Challenges/Barriers
Pulmonary disease	Still smoking, second-hand smoke exposure
Bowel disease	Poor diet, medication management
Diabetes control	Poor diet, inadequate exercise
Kidney disease	Rigid dialysis schedule, side effects of medication, financial costs, family challenges
Cardiovascular disease	Financial costs, effectiveness/side effects of medication, medication management
Hypertension	Disbelief that medication is effective, side effects of medication
Drug and alcohol addiction/treatment	Co-occurring health issues (hepatitis C, HIV, etc.), relapse, legal issues, transportation issues, employment barriers, relational issues, medication adherence
Smoking	Cravings, withdrawal, relapse, cost/funding needed for nicotine replacement therapy, mood issues due to withdrawal
HIV	Side effects of medication, rigid medication schedule
Mental health disorders	Side effects of medication, medication management, attending appointments, lack of health insurance, cost of medications, cost of appointments
Cancer prevention/ treatment	Inability to pay for screening/treatment, health insurance coverage concerns, inability to leave work, fear of diagnosis/mortality, coexisting/comorbid illness, caregiving demands, treatment side effects, cost of medications

"Good morning, Mrs. Jones. My name is _____, and I am your Patient Navigator.

At this clinic, Patient Navigators assist patients with life problems and stressful issues that sometimes get in the way of receiving your treatment and other types of health care.

I will help you with solving some of these problems and helping you cope with your new treatment regimen. I often see other women, just like you who have experiences similar to yours.

I will see you every other day when you come in for your treatment and will call you to follow up and remind you of your appointments. You can contact me or tell your nurse you'd like to see me, as well. I work M-F during the day and on-call in the evenings, but there is another patient navigator here in the clinic during the weekends. You can also leave me a message. Here is my card with my contact information.

Do you mind if I spend some time talking with you, getting to know you, and ask you some questions?"

Figure 2.4 Structuring Your Introduction

The relational component is essentially what MI is grounded on—the "spirit" of MI. This interpersonal spirit of MI involves engaging with the woman and developing rapport. To secure a trusting relationship throughout your work together, developing rapport is critical to gathering information. It is important to remain respectful, collaborative, and empathic not only throughout each conversation but also over the course of the relationship. Building rapport can begin with your first visit when you introduce yourself. This introduction should explain who you are, your role, why you are seeing your patient (with normalizing language), what to expect from subsequent visits, your availability, and the best way to reach you if needed. It is important to ask permission to spend some time getting to know her by talking (Figure 2.4).

For instance, if you are trying to encourage your patient to seek mammogram screening, your introductory conversation could consist of the following:

1. Ask for permission to discuss breast cancer and mammogram screening.
2. Ask what she already knows about breast cancer and mammogram screening.
3. Ask for permission to educate her about the risk of delayed diagnosis and importance of early screening.

It is important to be supportive by identifying where the patient is in the process of getting screening by asking permission. If we minimize or ignore where the patient is in this process, we are going to lose her pretty quickly. And often, she will tell you that she is satisfied and thank you for doing a great job of helping her. If she is not ready to get her mammogram screening, she will likely let you know. Some of the relational components might overlap with process skill development, which is discussed in Module 1.3 in this volume.

Reminder Checklist

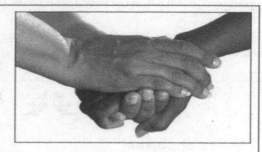

Figure 2.5 Am I Engaging the Right Way?

You can use the questions in Figure 2.5 to ensure that you are doing your best to properly engage with your patient.

One of the best-known technical components of MI is OARS: Open-ended questions, Affirmations, Reflective listening, and Summarizing. These four core MI skills are important in helping women overcome their barriers so they can attend to their health.

- *Open-ended questions* are those that cannot be answered with a "yes" or a "no." It is not always wrong to ask a "closed" question, but it is best to use many more open questions than closed ones.
- *Affirmations* are statements of support that point out the patient's strengths and positive aspects, delivered in a genuine manner. Affirmations differ from praise in that they have more depth than simply saying, "That's great."
- *Reflective listening* involves responding to your patient in ways that show you have listened to her carefully and understand what she is saying, often at a slightly deeper level than what the patient actually said. You can think of these statements as guessing at the meaning by reflecting back what the patient said, in an expanded manner. One way to practice doing this is to stop talking! You cannot build skill at listening if you are constantly speaking. If you are talking, you are not listening. This rule also applies to talking inside your mind as your patient is speaking. If you are thinking about the next thing that you want to say, you are not listening intently to what is being said.
- *Summarizing* involves collecting two or three ideas that the patient said and organizing the information in order to move the conversation forward. Summaries link things that have been said by noticing patterns or themes in what the patient is saying. Select significant statements throughout the conversation, and then summarize them. This reinforces the idea for the patient through hearing it again

during that summary. This not only ensures that you understand but also shows your patient that you are actively listening to her.

Figure 2.6 lists examples of OARS statements specifically for the cancer care of low-income women of color.

Open-ended questions:

- "How can I assist you today?"
- "What are some of your concerns about receiving radiation?"
- "How might your family assist you while you go to your chemotherapy appointment?"

Affirmations:

- "Although you sound like you may not be interested in getting a colonoscopy now, I appreciate you making it to this appointment today and taking the time to talk with me today."
- "Getting to work is hard because of your problems with transportation, but you've been able to hold a steady job for the past year."
- "Your commitment to your family is clear by the ways in which you care for your children."

Reflections:

- "It seems like there are parts of the radiation therapy that you would not like to go through."
- "What matters most to you is that you are still able to provide for your family."

Summarizing:

- "Let me see if I've got this so far. It sounds like you are feeling more positive about having the mammogram now. Several months ago, you couldn't have done it, but now that you have started to have your mom watch your daughter, you are ready to do it. I understand that it's really important—maybe even critical—for you to care for your family first. It's who you are. Is this accurate?"
- "I'd like to review what we've talked about so far, to be sure I'm understanding you correctly. Your primary concerns about having a Pap screening are about the logistics of getting time off of work, finding childcare, and being able to pay for the exam. Is that correct?"

Figure 2.6 OARS

Behavioral Skills

Behavioral skills should be coupled with the three skills we have already discussed—overcoming barriers, providing tailored educational information, and using motivational skills—to enhance patient navigation and thus help improve adherence to cancer care.

Behavioral skills are critical determinants of health that influence whether well-informed and well-motivated individuals are capable of carrying out a health behavior effectively (Fisher & Fisher, 2000; Fisher et al., 2002, 2006). A focus on behavioral skills during patient navigation involves concrete and practical tasks needed to prepare for cancer care, usually care related to screening or treatment.

Behavioral skills can be categorized into systematic skills and procedural skills. *Systematic skills* involve the logistics of getting into cancer care (e.g., the number to call to get screening, where to go, the days and hours in which screenings are scheduled, insurance co-pay information, how to obtain an appointment at the clinic, following up on scheduled appointments, unforeseen scheduling challenges, if transportation is provided) (Carrasquillo et al., 2018). *Procedural skills* involve how to prepare for the actual procedure (e.g., what to expect during the screening procedure, what to do or avoid doing to prepare for the screening appointment, questions to ask the provider during the appointment). Figure 2.7 provides recommended behavioral skill guidelines for mammogram screening and Papanicolaou (Pap) testing. Behavioral skills requires more active involvement in care by asking more appropriate and relevant questions, thus helping to improve one's self-efficacy (Raich et al., 2012). Self-efficacy has been incorporated in the health behavior models and has been shown to correlate to behavioral uptake (Jandorf et al., 2013). Thus, having systematic and procedural skill knowledge, exhibited through strong behavioral skills, gives a woman the confidence to act and behave on recommended cancer care.

Adapting Patient Navigation

There is scant research investigating the use of theory-based behavioral frameworks for interventions to help improve adherence among high-risk, hard-to-reach populations. However, Information-Motivation-Behavioral skills (IMB) is a well-known evidence-based adherence model that asserts that information, motivation, and behavioral skills are the fundamental determinants to screening behavior (Fisher & Fisher, 2000). IMB use and success has been documented in other behavior change interventions, like adherence to antiretroviral HIV/AIDS therapy, HIV risk prevention, diabetes self-care, and condom use among low-income women (Anderson et al., 2006; Fisher et al., 2002, 2006; Osborn & Egede, 2010). According to IMB, to the extent that women are well informed, are motivated to act, and possess behavioral skills required to act effectively, it is likely that they will behave favorably (e.g., initiate and maintain regular mammography). IMB serves as the theoretical guide for the adoption of an adapted model that improves upon classic patient navigation—Navigation Information-Motivation-Behavioral skills Problem solving (NIMBs-Ps)—by adding (1) working to overcome barriers and (2) expanding patient navigation. Thus, the NIMBs-Ps model asserts that, in combination with "barrier-reduction" patient navigation techniques, information, motivation,

How to Prepare for Your Mammogram

- If you can, choose a facility that specializes in mammograms and does many mammograms a day.
- Going to the same facility for your mammogram every time will allow for easy comparison of your mammograms from year to year.
- Bring a list of the places and dates of mammograms, biopsies, or other breast treatments you've had before if this is your first time at a particular facility.
- If you've had mammograms at another facility, try to get those records to bring with you to the new facility (or have them sent) so the old pictures can be compared to the new ones.
- Schedule your mammogram when your breasts are not tender or swollen to help reduce discomfort and get better pictures. Try to avoid the week just before your period.
- Reduce your intake of caffeinated drinks and chocolate for three to four days before the exam, as caffeine can increase benign lumps and lead to greater discomfort during breast compressions.
- Don't wear deodorant, antiperspirant, powder, or skin lotion on the day you go for the exam. These products sometimes contain substances that can show up on the screening results as white spots. Consider bringing deodorant or other necessary products with you to put on after the exam if you are not planning to go home afterward.
- It may be more convenient to wear a two-piece outfit, so you'll only need to remove your top and bra for the exam.
- You may decide to take one or two tablets of ibuprofen or acetaminophen about an hour before your appointment.
- Tell your healthcare provider about any recent changes or problems in your breasts before getting the mammogram.

How to Prepare for Your Pap Screening

- Tell your doctor if you're menstruating, as it may affect your results. If you can, try to schedule your Pap test for at least 5 days after the end of your period. A Pap test can be performed during your period, but it is better to schedule the test for another time.
- Avoid having intercourse, douching, or using spermicidal products for two to three days before the test. Most medical professionals advise against douching for any reason. You should not put anything in or around your vagina to clean it, other than soap and water on the outside of your vagina/vulva.
- Avoid using tampons, birth control foams, vaginal medicines, douches, and vaginal creams and powders for two to three days before the test in order to avoid washing away abnormal cells.
- Try to relax, stay calm, and breathe deeply. This will help make the procedure easier and more comfortable for you.

Figure 2.7 Preparation Tips

Cancer.net. (2018). Pap test. https://www.cancer.net/navigating-cancer-care/diagnosing-cancer/tests-and-procedures/pap-test and Healthline Medical Review Team. (2019). Pap smear (Pap test): What to expect. https://www.healthline.com/health/pap-smear#preparation

behavioral skills, and problem solving are the fundamental determinants of behavior (e.g., screening, diagnostic test, or treatment).

Figure 2.8 shows these adaptations to the traditional IMB model. This figure illustrates the interrelationships among the relevant NIMBs-Ps constructs and operations used to translate into an evidence-based mammography intervention. For example, for an low-income unscreened woman, barrier-reduction navigation activities (often providing needed social service resources and referrals), combined with problem solving, might be needed first (and throughout) to address her daily stressors, practical issues, and circumstances. As we noted earlier, studies show that for those living in poverty, meeting basic human needs is perceived as more important than obtaining cancer prevention and screening (Bell et al., 2017; Wells et al., 2019). Thus, both information and motivation, along with problem-solving techniques, are needed to advance interest in learning systematic and procedural behavioral skills. This means that well-informed individuals are not necessarily motivated to engage in cancer screening behaviors and motivated individuals are not necessarily well informed about screening practices. In fact, information, problem solving, and motivation act as tools to develop behavioral skill activation, which is an additional critical determinant of whether people would be capable of cancer care behavioral uptake.

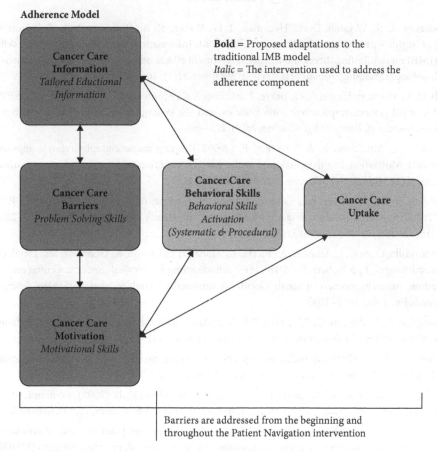

Figure 2.8 Navigation-Information-Motivation-Behavioral skills—Problem solving (NIMBs-Ps) conceptual model.

Conclusion

Improving cancer screening and diagnostic follow-up is essential for reducing cancer incidence and mortality, particularly in low-income women of color, where the greatest disparities exist. Addressing these disparities is best accomplished with community partnerships. Peer community health navigators (CHNs), who are survivors or women of color who have had personal experience with cancer and are familiar with the community, are helpful because they can identify with the issue and eliminate some of the trust issues that exist for this population. The use of evidence-based clinical interventions (NIMBs-Ps) extended within a community-engaged research (CEnR) context is a paradigm shift from traditional patient navigation models of cancer prevention and control. This can be impactful because it has the potential to inform future patient navigation interventions in the area of cancer prevention and control by use of empirically supported clinical behavior change techniques and principles, within a community context. Patient navigation services should not be solely imbedded and constrained within the traditional clinical healthcare system. This chapter fills a substantial gap in our knowledge of how interventions make it into the real-world CEnR and practice.

References

Anderson, E. S., Wagstaff, D. A., Heckman, T. G., Winett, R. A., Roffman, R. A., Solomon, L. J., Cargill, V., Kelly, J. A., & Sikkema, K. J. (2006). Information-motivation-behavioral skills (IMB) model: Testing direct and mediated treatment effects on condom use among women in low-income housing. *Annals of Behavioral Medicine, 31*(1), 70–79.

Bell, H. S., Martínez-Hume, A. C., Baker, A. M., Elwell, K., Montemayor, I., & Hunt, L. M. (2017). Medicaid reform, responsibilization policies, and the synergism of barriers to low-income health-seeking. *Human Organization, 76*(3), 275–286.

Bernstein, J., Mutschler, P., & Bernstein, E. (2000). Keeping mammography referral appointments: Motivation, health beliefs, and access barriers experienced by older minority women. *Journal of Midwifery & Women's Health, 45*(4), 308–313.

Calhoun, E. A., Whitley, E. M., Esparza, A., Ness, E., Greene, A., Garcia, R., & Valverde, P. A. (2010). A national patient navigator training program. *Health Promotion Practice, 11*(2), 205–215. doi:10.1177/1524839908323521

Carrasquillo, O., Seay, J., Amofah, A., Pierre, L., Alonzo, Y., McCann, S., Gonzalez, M., Trevil, D., Koru-Sengul, T., & Kobetz, E. (2018). HPV self-sampling for cervical cancer screening among ethnic minority women in south Florida: A randomized trial. *Journal of General Internal Medicine, 33*(7), 1077–1083.

Champion, V. L., & Scott, C. R. (1997). Reliability and validity of breast cancer screening belief scales in African American women. *Nursing Research, 46*, 331–337.

Diclemente, C. C. (2010). Mindfulness specific or generic mechanisms of action. *Addiction, 105*(10), 1707–1708. doi:10.1111/j.1360-0443.2010.03013.x

Ell, K., Bin, X., Wells, A., Nedjat-Haiem, F., Lee, P. J., & Vourlekis, B. (2008). Economic stress among low-income women with cancer: Effects on quality of life. *Cancer, 112*(3), 616–625.

Ell, K., & Wells, A. (2006). Adapted problem solving therapy for primary care: Maintenance group manual and program protocol. Multifaceted diabetes and depression program (MDDP) and alleviating depression among patients with cancer (ADAPt-C) clinical trials.

Ferrante, J. M., Chen, P. H., & Kim, S. (2007). The effect of patient navigation on time to diagnosis, anxiety, and satisfaction in urban minority women with abnormal mammograms: A randomized controlled trial. *Journal of Urban Health, 85*(1), 114–124.

Fisher, J. D., & Fisher, W. A. (2000). *Theoretical approaches to individual-level change in HIV risk behavior*. Centre for Health, Information and Prevention Documents. Paper 4. http://digitalcommons.uconn.edu/chip_docs/4

Fisher, J. D., Fisher, W. A., Amico, K. R., & Harman, J. J. (2006). An information-motivation-behavioral skills model of adherence to antiretroviral therapy. *Health Psychology, 25*(4), 462–473.

Fisher, J. D., Fisher, W. A., Bryan, A. D., & Stephen, J. M. (2002). Information-motivation-behavioral skills model-based HIV risk behavior change intervention for inner-city high school youth. *Health Psychology, 21*(2), 177–186. doi:10.1037/0278-6133.21.2.177

Freeman, H. P. (2006). Patient navigation: A community-centered approach to reducing cancer mortality. *Journal of Cancer Education, 21*(1), S11–S14.

Freeman, H. P., & Rodriguez, R. L. (2011). The history and principles of patient navigation. *Cancer, 117*(15), 3539–3542.

Heppner, P. P., Witty, T. E., & Dixon, W. A. (2004). Problem-solving appraisal and human adjustment: A review of 20 years of research using the Problem Solving Inventory. *Counseling Psychologist, 32*(3), 344–428. https://doi.org/10.1177/0011000003262793

Hopkins, J., & Mumber, M. P. (2009). Patient navigation through the cancer care continuum: An overview. *Journal of Oncology Practice, 5*(4), 150–152.

Howard, A. F., Balneaves, L. G., & Bottorff, J. L. (2007). Ethnocultural women's experiences of breast cancer: A qualitative meta-study. *Cancer Nursing, 30*(4), E27–E35.

Hunt, B. R., Allgood, K. L., Kanoon, J. M., & Benjamins, M. R. (2017). Keys to the successful implementation of community-based outreach and navigation: Lessons from a breast health navigation program. *Journal of Cancer Education, 32*(1), 175–182.

Jandorf, L., Braschi, C., Ernstoff, E., Wong, C. R., Thelemaque, L., Winkel, G., Thompson, H. S., Redd, W. H., & Itzkowitz, S. H. (2013). Culturally targeted patient navigation for increasing African Americans' adherence to screening colonoscopy: A randomized clinical trial. *Cancer Epidemiology, Biomarkers & Prevention, 22*(9), 1577–1587. doi:10.1158/1055-9965. EPI-12-1275

Kreuter, M. W., & McClure, S. M. (2004). The role of culture in health communication. *Annual review of public health, 25*, 439–455.

Kreuter, M. W., McQueen, A., Boyum, S., & Fu, Q. (2016). Unmet basic needs and health intervention effectiveness in low-income populations. *Preventive Medicine, 91*, 70–75. https://doi.org/10.1016/j.ypmed.2016.08.006

Lopez, V. A., & Castro, F. G. (2006). Participation and program outcomes in a Church-based cancer prevention program for Hispanic women. *Journal of Community Health, 31*(4), 343–362. https://doi.org/10.1007/s10900-006-9016-6

Lobb, R., & Colditz, G. A. (2013). Implementation science and its application to population health. *Annual Review of Public Health, 34*, 235–251. doi:10.1146/annurev-pubhealth-031912-114444

McKenney, K. M., Martinez, N. G., & Yee, L. M. (2018). Patient navigation across the spectrum of women's health care in the United States. *American Journal of Obstetrics & Gynecology, 218*(3), 280–286.

Miller, W. R., & Rollnick, S. (2012). *Motivational interviewing: Helping people change* (3rd ed.). Guilford Press.

Nezu, A. M., Nezu, C. M., & Houts, P. S. (1994). *Coping with cancer: A problem-solving approach.* Paper presented at the International Congress of Behavioral Medicine, Amsterdam, the Netherlands.

Osborn, C. Y., & Egede, L. E. (2010). Validation of an information-motivation-behavioral skills model of diabetes self-care (IMB-DSC). *Patient Education and Counseling, 79*(1), 49–54.

Parker, V. A., Clark, J. A., Leyson, J., Calhoun, E., Carroll, J. K., Freund, K. M., & Battaglia, T. A. (2010). Patient navigation: Development of a protocol for describing what navigators do. *Health Services Research, 45*(2), 514–531. doi:10.1111/j.1475-6773.2009.01079.x

Paskett, E. D., McLaughlin, J. M., Lehman, A. M., Katz, M. L., Tatum, C. M., & Oliveri, J. M. (2011). Evaluating the efficacy of lay health advisors for increasing risk-appropriate Pap test screening: A randomized controlled trial among Ohio Appalachian women. *Cancer Epidemiology, Biomarkers & Prevention, 20*(5), 835–843. doi:10.1158/1055-9965.EPI-10-0880

Pedersen, A., & Hack, T. F. (2010). Pilots of oncology health care: A concept analysis of the patient navigator role. *Oncology Nursing Forum, 37*(1), 55–60.

Percac-Lima, S., Grant, R. W., Green, A. R., Ashburner, J. M., Gamba, G., Oo, S., Richter, J. M., & Atlas, S. J. (2008). A culturally tailored navigator program for colorectal cancer screening in a community health center: A randomized, controlled trial. *Journal of General Internal Medicine, 24*(2), 211–217.

Pudkasam, S., Polman, R., Pitcher, M., Fisher, M., Chinlumprasert, N., Stojanovska, L., & Apostolopoulos, V. (2018). Physical activity and breast cancer survivors: Importance of adherence, motivational interviewing, and psychological health. *Maturitas, 116*, 66–72. doi:10.1016/j.maturitas.2018.07.010

Raich, P. C., Whitley, E. M., Thorland, W., Valverde, P., Fairclough, D., & Denver Patient Navigation Research Program. (2012). Patient navigation improves cancer diagnostic resolution: An individually randomized clinical trial in an underserved population. *Cancer Epidemiology, Biomarkers & Prevention, 21*(10), 1629–1638. doi:10.1158/1055-9965.EPI-12-0513

Ravenell, J., Thompson, H., Cole, H., Plumhoff, J., Cobb, G., Afolabi, L., Boutin-Foster, C., Wells, M., Scott, M., & Ogedegbe, G. (2013). A novel community-based study to address disparities in hypertension and colorectal cancer: A study protocol for a randomized control trial. *Trials, 14*(287), 1–13.

Russell, K. M., Monahan, P., Wagle, A., & Champion, V. (2007). Differences in health and cultural beliefs by stage of mammography screening adoption in African American women. *Cancer, 109*(2 Suppl), 386–395. doi:10.1002/cncr.22359

Shelton, R. C., Thompson, H. S., Jandorf, L., Varela, A., Oliveri, B., Villagra, C., Valdimarsdottir, H. B., & Redd, W. H. (2011). Training experiences of lay and professional patient navigators for colorectal cancer screening. *Journal of Cancer Education, 26*, 277–284. doi:10.1007/s13187-010 0185-8

Skinner, C. S., Strecher, V. J., & Hospers, H. (1994). Physician's recommendations for mammography: Do tailored messages make a difference? *American Journal of Public Health, 84*(1), 43–49.

Tatum, A. K., & Houston, E. (2017). Examining the interplay between depression, motivation, and antiretroviral therapy adherence: A social cognitive approach. *AIDS Care, 29*(3), 306–310.

University of Washington. (2019). Problem solving treatment. https://aims.uw.edu/collaborative-care/behavioral-interventions/problem-solving-treatment-pst

Vargas, R. B., Ryan, G. W., Jackson, C. A., Rodriguez, R., & Freeman, H. P. (2008). Characteristics of the original patient navigation programs to reduce disparities in the diagnosis and treatment of breast cancer. *Cancer, 113*(2), 426–433.

Wells, A., Gulbas, L., Sanders-Thompson, V., Shon, E.J., & Kreuter, M. (2013). African American breast cancer survivors participating in a support group: Translating research into oncology practice, *Journal of Cancer Education*. doi: 10.1007/s13187-013-0592-8

Wells, A. A., Palinkas, L. A., Williams, S. L., & Ell, K. (2015). Retaining low-income minority cancer patients in a depression treatment intervention trial: Lessons learned. *Community Mental Health Journal, 51*(6), 715–722.

Wells, A. A., Sanders Thompson, V. L., Ross, W., Camp Yeakey, C., & Notaro, S. (2019). *Poverty and place: Cancer prevention among low-income women of color.* Lexington Books.

Wells, A. A., Shon, E., McGowan, K., & James, A. (2017). Perspectives of low-income African-American women non-adherent to mammography screening: The importance of information, behavioral skills, and motivation. *Journal of Cancer Education, 32*(2), 328–334.

Wells, K. J., Battaglia, T. A., Dudley, D. J., Garcia, R., Greene, A., Calhoun, E., Mandelblatt, J. S., Paskett, E. D., & Raich, P. C. (2008). Patient navigation: State of the art or is it science? *Cancer, 113*(8), 1999–2010.

Wells, K. J., Meade, C. D., Calcano, E., Lee, J., Rivers, D., & Roetzheim, R. G. (2011). Innovative approaches to reducing cancer health disparities. *Journal of Cancer Education, 26*(4), 649–657.

Yosha, A. M., Carroll, J. K., Hendren, S., Salamone, C. M., Sanders, M., Fiscella, K., & Epstein, R. M. (2011). Patient navigation from the paired perspectives of cancer patients and navigators: A qualitative analysis. *Patient Education and Counseling, 82*(3), 396–401.

Suggested Reading

Allicock, M., Kaye, L., Johnson, L., Carr, C., Alick, C., Gellin, M., & Campbell, M. (2012). The use of motivational interviewing to promote peer-to-peer support for cancer survivors. *Clinical Journal of Oncology Nursing, 16*(5), E156–E163.

Altekruse, S. F., Kosary, C. L., & Krapcho, M. (2010). *SEER cancer statistics review, 1975–2007.* National Cancer Institute.

Ashing-Giwa, K. T. (1999). Quality of life and psychosocial outcomes in long-term survivors of breast cancer: A focus on African-American women. *Journal of Psychosocial Oncology, 17*(3/4), 47–62.

Ashing-Giwa, K. T., George, M., & Jones, V. (2018). Health-related quality of life and care satisfaction outcomes: Informing psychosocial oncology care among Latina and African American young breast cancer survivors. *Psycho-Oncology, 27*(4), 1213–1220.

Ashing-Giwa, K. T., Padilla, G., Tejero, J., Kraemer, J., Wright, K., Coscarelli, A., Clayton, S., Williams, I., & Hills, D. (2004). Understanding the breast cancer experience of women: A qualitative study of African American, Asian American, Latina and Caucasian cancer survivors. *Psycho-Oncology, 13*, 408–428.

Auslander, W., & Freedenthal, S. (2006). Social work and chronic disease: Diabetes, heart disease, and HIV/AIDS. In S. Gehlert & T. A. Browne (Eds.), *Handbook of health social work*. John Wiley & Sons, Inc., 532–567.

Barkhof, E., Meijer, C., de Sonneville, L., Linszen, D., & de Haan, L. (2013). The effect of motivational interviewing on medication adherence and hospitalization rates in nonadherent patients with multi-episode schizophrenia. *Schizophrenia Bulletin, 39*(6), 1242–1251. doi:10.1093/schbul/sbt138

Beckjord, E. B., & Klassen, A. C. (2008). Cultural values and secondary prevention of breast cancer in African American women. *Cancer Control, 15*(1), 63–71.

Bernard, V., Howe, W., Royalty, J., Helsel, W., Kammerer, W., & Richardson, L. (2012). Timeliness of cervical cancer diagnosis and initiation of treatment in the National Breast and Cervical Cancer Early Detection Program. *Journal of Women's Health*, 21, 776–782.

Beverly, L., Yoo, G. J., & Levine, E. G. (2014). "Trust in the Lord": Religious and spiritual practices of African American breast cancer survivors. *Journal of Religion and Health*, 53(6), 1706–1716.

Bibb, S. C. G. (2001). The relationship between access and stage at diagnosis of breast cancer in African American and Caucasian women. *Oncology Nursing Forum*, 28(4), 711–719.

Blumer, H. (1954). What is wrong with social theory? *American Sociological Review*, 19(1), 3.

Boeije, H. (2002). A purposeful approach to the constant comparative method in the analysis of qualitative interviews. *Quality & Quantity*, 36, 391–409.

Bondy, M. L., & Newman, L. A. (2000). Breast cancer risk assessment models: Applicability to African American women. *Cancer*, 97(S1), 230–235.

Borchelt, G. (2018). The impact poverty has on women's health. American Bar Association. https://www.americanbar.org/groups/crsj/publications/human_rights_magazine_home/the-state-of-healthcare-in-the-united-states/poverty-on-womens-health/

Bourjolly, J. N. (1998). Differences in religiousness among Black and White women with breast cancer. *Social Work in Health Care*, 28(1), 21–39.

Bourjolly, J. N., Barg, F. K., & Hirschman, K. B. (2003). African-American and white women's appraisal of their breast cancer. *Journal of Psychosocial Oncology*, 21(3), 43–61.

Bourjolly, J. N., & Hirschman, K. B. (2001). Similarities in coping strategies but differences in sources of support among African American and White women coping with breast cancer. *Journal of Psychosocial Oncology*, 19(2), 17–38.

Boutin-Foster, C., Scott, E., Rodriguez, A., Ramos, R., Kanna, B., Michelen, W., Charlson, M., & Ogedegbe, G. (2013). The Trial Using Motivational Interviewing and Positive Affect and Self-Affirmation in African-Americans with Hypertension (TRIUMPH): From theory to clinical trial implementation. *Contemporary Clinical Trials*, 35(1), 8–14. doi:10.1016/j.cct.2013.02.002

Boyd, A. S., & Wilmoth, M. C. (2006). An innovative community-based intervention for African American women with breast cancer: The Witness Project. *Health & Social Work*, 31(1), 77–80.

Bradley, P. K. (2005). The delay and worry experience of African American women with breast cancer. *Oncology Nursing Forum*, 32(2), 243–249.

Brodie, D., Inoue, A., & Shaw, D. (2008). Motivational interviewing to change quality of life for people with chronic heart failure: A randomised controlled trial. *International Journal of Nursing Studies*, 45(4), 489–500.

Campbell, C., Craig, J., Eggert, J., & Bailey-Dorton, C. (2010). Implementing and measuring the impact of patient navigation at a comprehensive community cancer center. *Oncology Nursing Forum*, 37(1), 61–68.

Campbell, M., Carr, C., DeVellis, B., Switzer, B., Biddle, A., Amamoo, M. M., Walsh, J., Zhou, B., & Sandler, R. (2009). A randomized trial of tailoring and motivational interviewing to promote fruit and vegetable consumption for cancer prevention and control. *Annals of Behavioral Medicine*, 38(2), 71–85. doi:10.1007/s12160-009-9140-5

Caplan, L. S., & Helzlsouer, K. J. (1992-1993). Delay in breast cancer: A review of the literature. *Public Health Reviews*, 20(3-4), 187–214.

Carroll, J. K., Humiston, S. G., Meldrum, S., Salamone, C. M., Jean-Pierre, P., Epstein, R. M., & Fiscella, K. (2010). Patients' experiences with navigation for cancer care. *Patient Education and Counseling*, 80(2), 241–247.

Chen, S., Creedy, D., Lin, H., & Wollin, J. (2012). Effects of motivational interviewing intervention on self-management, psychological and glycemic outcomes in type 2 diabetes: A randomized controlled trial. *International Journal of Nursing Studies, 49*(6), 637–644.

Christensen, A. J., & Johnson, J. A. (2002). Patient adherence with medical treatment regimens: An interactive approach. *Current Directions in Psychological Science, 11*(3), 94–97.

Collins, T., Stradtman, L. R., Vanderpool, R. C., Neace, D. R., & Cooper, K. D. (2015). A community-academic partnership to increase Pap testing in Appalachian Kentucky. *American Journal of Preventive Medicine, 49*(2), 324–330.

Conway-Phillips, R., & Millon-Underwood, S. (2009). Breast cancer screening behaviors of African American women: A comprehensive review, analysis, and critique of nursing research. *Association of Black Nursing Faculty, 20,* 97–101.

Cooper, L. (2012). Combined motivational interviewing and cognitive-behavioral therapy with older adult drug and alcohol abusers. *Health & Social Work, 37*(3), 173–179.

Copeland, V. C., Scholle, S. H., & Binko, J. A. (2003). Patient satisfaction: African American women's views of the patient-doctor relationship. *Journal of Health & Social Policy, 17*(2), 35–48.

Creswell, J. W., & Maietta, R. C. (2002). Qualitative research. In D. C. Miller & N. J. Salkind (Eds.), *Handbook of research design and social measurement* (6th ed., pp. 143–184). Sage Publications.

Culver, J. L., Arena, P. L., Antoni, M. H., & Carver, C. S. (2002). Coping and distress among women under treatment for early stage breast cancer: Comparing African Americans, Hispanics and non-Hispanic Whites. *Psycho-Oncology, 11,* 495–504.

Davis, C. M., Nyamathi, A. M., Abuatiq, A., Fike, G. C., & Wilson, A. M. (2018). Understanding supportive care factors among African American breast cancer survivors. *Journal of Transcultural Nursing, 29*(1), 21–29.

Dohan, D., & Schrag, D. (2005). Using navigators to improve care of underserved patients. *Cancer, 104*(4), 848–855.

Duncan, V. J., Parrott, R. L., & Silk, K. J. (2001). African American women's perceptions of the role of genetics in breast cancer risk. *American Journal of Health Studies* (Special Issue: "The Health of Women of Color"), *17*(2), 50–58.

Efraimsson, E., Fossum, B., Ehrenberg, A., Larsson, K., & Klang, B. (2012). Use of motivational interviewing in smoking cessation at nurse-led chronic obstructive pulmonary disease clinics. *Journal of Advanced Nursing, 68*(4), 767–782. doi:10.1111/j.1365-2648.2011.05766.x

Ell, K., Quon, B., Quinn, D. I., Dwight-Johnson, M., Wells, A., & Lee, P. (2007). Improving treatment of depression among low-income patients with cancer: The design of the ADAPt-C study. *General Hospital Psychiatry, 29*(3), 223–231.

Ell, K., Vourlekis, B., Xie, B., Nedjat-Haiem, F. R., Lee, P. J., Muderspach, L., Russell, C., & Palinkas, L. A. (2009). Cancer treatment adherence among low-income women with breast or gynecologic cancer. *Cancer, 115*(19), 4606–4615.

Flannery, I. M., Yoo, G. J., & Levine, E. G. (2019). Keeping us all whole: Acknowledging the agency of African American breast cancer survivors and their systems of social support. *Supportive Care in Cancer, 27*(7), 2625–2632.

Flickinger, T. E., Rose, G., Wilson, I. B., Wolfe, H., Saha, S., Korthuis, P., Massa, M., Berry, S., Barton Laws, M., Sharp, V., Moore, R. D., & Beach, M. C. (2013). Motivational interviewing by HIV care providers is associated with patient intentions to reduce unsafe sexual behavior. *Patient Education & Counseling, 93*(1), 122–129. doi:10.1016/j.pec.2013.04.001

Fowler, B. A. (2006a). Claiming health: Mammography screening decision making of African American women. *Oncology Nursing Forum, 33*(5), 969–975.

Fowler, B. A. (2006b). Social processes used by African American women in making decisions about mammography screening. *Journal of Nursing Scholarship*, *38*(3), 247–254.

Fukui, S., Kugaya, A., Okamura, H., Kamiya, M., Koike, M., Nakanishi, T., Imoto, S., Kanagawa, K., & Uchitomi, Y. (2000). A psychosocial group prevention for Japanese women with primary breast carcinoma: A randomized controlled trial. *Cancer*, *89*(5), 1026–1036.

Gabram, S., Lund, M. J., Gardner, J., Hatchett, N., Bumpers, H. L., Okoli, J., Rizzo, M., Johnson, B. J., Kirkpatrick, G. B., & Brawley, O. W. (2008). Effects of an outreach and internal navigation program on breast cancer diagnosis in an urban cancer center with a large African-American population. *Cancer*, *113*(3), 602–607.

García-Llana, H., Remor, E., del Peso, G., Celadilla, O., & Selgas, R. (2014). Motivational interviewing promotes adherence and improves wellbeing in pre-dialysis patients with advanced chronic kidney disease. *Journal of Clinical Psychology in Medical Settings*, *21*(1), 103–115. doi:10.1007/s10880-013-9383-y

Garfield, S. L. (1963). A note on patients' reasons for terminating therapy. *Psychological Reports*, *13*, 38.

Geertz, C. (1973). *The interpretation of cultures*. Basic Books.

Ghafoor, A., Jemal, A., Ward, E., Cokkinides, V., Smith, R., & Thun, M. (2003). Trends in breast cancer by race and ethnicity. *CA: A Journal for Clinicians*, *53*, 342–355.

Gibson, L. M., & Hendricks, C. S. (2006). Integrative review of spirituality in African American breast cancer survivors. *Association of Black Nursing Faculty Journal*, *17*(2), 67–72.

Givens, J. L., Datto, C. J., Ruckdeschel, K., Knott, K., Zubritsky, C., Oslin, D. W., Nyshadham, S., Vanguri, P., & Barg, F. K. (2006). Older patients' aversion to antidepressants: A qualitative study. *Journal of General Internal Medicine*, *21*(2), 146–151.

Glantz, K., Rimer, B. K., & Lewis, F. M. (Eds.) (2002). *Health behavior and health education* (3rd ed.). Jossey-Bass.

Glaser, B. G., & Strauss, A. L. (1967). *The discovery of grounded theory: Strategies for qualitative research*. Aldine de Gruyter.

Gunn, C. M., Parker, V. A., Bak, S. M., Ko, N., Nelson, K. P., & Battaglia, T. A. (2017). Social network structures of breast cancer patients and the contributing role of patient navigators. *The Oncologist*, *22*(8), 918–924.

Hahn, K. M., Bondy, M. L., & Selvan, M. (2007). Factors associated with advanced disease stage at diagnosis in a population-based study of patients with newly diagnosed breast cancer. *American Journal of Epidemiology*, *166*(9), 1035–1044.

Hall, I. J., Moorman, P. G., Millikan, R. C., & Newman, B. (2005). Comparative analysis of breast cancer risk factors among African-American women and white women. *American Journal of Epidemiology*, *161*(1), 40–51.

Hardcastle, S. J., Taylor, A. H., Bailey, M. P., Harley, R. A., & Hagger, M. S. (2013). Effectiveness of a motivational interviewing intervention on weight loss, physical activity and cardiovascular disease risk factors: A randomised controlled trial with a 12-month post-intervention follow-up. *International Journal of Behavioral Nutrition & Physical Activity*, *10*(1), 40–55. doi:10.1186/1479-5868-10-40

Heaton, J. (2008) Secondary analysis of qualitative data: An overview. *Historical Social Research*, *33*(3), 33–45.

Heiney, S. P., Gullatte, M., Hayne, P. D., Powe, B., & Habing, B. (2016). Fatalism revisited: Further psychometric testing across two studies. *Journal of Religion and Health*, *55*(4), 1472–1481.

Henderson, P. D., Gore, S. V., Davis, B. L., & Condon, E. H. (2003). African American women coping with breast cancer: A qualitative analysis. *Oncology Nursing Forum, 30*(4), 641–647.

Hendren, S., Griggs, J. J., Epstein, R. M., Carroll, J., Humiston, S., Rousseau, S., Jean-Pierre, P., Carroll, J., Yosha, A. M., Loader, S., & Fiscella, K. (2010). Study protocol: A randomized controlled trial of patient navigation-activation to reduce cancer health disparities. *BMC Cancer, 10*(1), 551.

Holland, J. C., Romano, S. J., Heilingenstein, J. H., Tepner, R. D., & Wilson, M. G. (1998). A controlled trial of fluoxetine and desipramine in depressed women with advanced cancer. *Psycho-Oncology, 7*(4), 291–300.

Holt, C. L., Kyles, A., Wiehagen, T., & Casey, C. (2003). Development of a spiritually based breast cancer education booklet for African American women. *Cancer Control, 10*(5), 37–44.

Holt, C. L., Lukwago, S. N., & Kreuter, M. (2003). Spirituality, breast cancer beliefs and mammography utilization among urban African American women. *Journal of Health Psychology, 8*(3), 383–396.

Horner, M. J., Alterkruse, S. F., Zou, Z., Wideroff, L., Katki, H. A., & Stinchcomb, D. G. (2011). U.S. geographic distribution of prevaccine era cervical cancer screening, incidence, stage, and mortality. *Cancer Epidemiology & Biomarkers, 20*, 591–599.

Jack, L. Jr., Airhihenbuwa, C. O., Murphy, F., Thompson-Reid, P., Wheatley, B., & Dickson-Smith, J. (1993). Cancer among low-income African-Americans: Implications for culture and community-based health promotion. *Wellness Perspectives, 9*(4), 57–68.

Jancin, B. (2004, February). Socioeconomics don't explain racial differences in breast cancer outcome. *Family Practice News, 34*(3), 64.

Jandorf, L., Gutierrez, Y., Lopez, J., Christie, J., & Itzkowitz, S. H. (2005). Use of a patient navigator to increase colorectal cancer screening in an urban neighborhood health clinic. *Journal of Urban Health, 82*(2), 216–224.

Jones, B. A., Patterson, E. A., & Calvocoressi, L. (2003). Mammography screening in African American women: Evaluating the research. *Cancer, 97*(S1), 258–272.

Jones, D. P. (2015). Knowledge, beliefs, and feelings about breast cancer: The perspective of African American women. *ABNF Journal, 26*(1), 5–10.

Kim, J. H., Menon, U., Wang, E., & Szalacha, L. (2010). Assessing the effects of culturally relevant intervention on breast cancer knowledge, beliefs, and mammography use among Korean American women. *Journal of Immigrant and Minority Health, 12*(4), 586–597.

Klassen, A. C., & Washington, C. (2008). How does social integration influence breast cancer control among urban African-American women? Results from a cross-sectional survey. *BMC Women's Health, 8*, 4.

Kleinman, A., Eisenberg, L., & Good, B. (1978). Culture, illness and care: Clinical lessons from anthropologic and cross-cultural research. *Annals of Internal Medicine, 88*, 251–258.

Koh, H. K., Judge, C. M., Ferrer, B., & Gershman, S. T. (2005). Using public health data systems to understand and eliminate cancer disparities. *Cancer Causes and Control, 16*, 15–26.

Korcha, R. A., Polcin, D. L., Evans, K., Bond, J. C., & Galloway, G. P. (2014). Intensive motivational interviewing for women with concurrent alcohol problems and methamphetamine dependence. *Journal of Substance Abuse Treatment, 46*(2), 113–119. doi:10.1016/j.jsat.2013.08.013

Lakerveld, J., Bot, S. D., Chinapaw, M. J., van Tulder, M. W., Kostense, P. J., Dekker, J. M., & Nijpels, G. (2013). Motivational interviewing and problem solving treatment to reduce type 2 diabetes and cardiovascular disease risk in real life: A randomized controlled trial. *International Journal of Behavioral Nutrition & Physical Activity, 10*(1), 47–55. doi:10.1186/1479-5868-10-47

Lasser, K. E., Murillo, J., Lisboa, S., Casimir, A. N., Valley-Shah, L., Emmons, K. M., Fletcher, R. H., & Ayanian, J. Z. (2011). Colorectal cancer screening among ethnically diverse, low-income patients. *Archives of Internal Medicine, 171*(10), 906–912.

Legler, J., Meissner, H. I., Coyne, C., Breen, N., Chollette, V., & Rimer, B. K. (2002). The effectiveness of interventions to promote mammography among women with historically lower rates of screening. *Cancer Epidemiology, Biomarkers, and Prevention, 11*(1), 59–71.

Lovejoy, T. I., & Heckman, T. G. (2014). Telephone-administered motivational interviewing and behavioral skills training to reduce risky sexual behavior in HIV-positive late middle-age and older adults. *Cognitive and Behavioral Practice, 21*(2), 224–236. doi:10.1016/j.cbpra.2013.10.003

Lucas Baker, J., Rodgers, C. R. R., Davis, Z. M., Gracely, E., & Bowleg, L. (2014). Results from a secondary data analysis regarding satisfaction with health care among African American women living with HIV/AIDS. *Journal of Obstetric, Gynecologic & Neonatal Nursing, 43*(5), 664–676.

Ma, C., Zhou, Y., Zhou, W., & Huang, C. (2014). Evaluation of the effect of motivational interviewing counseling on hypertension care. *Patient Education & Counseling, 95*(2), 231–237. doi:10.1016/j.pec.2014.01.011

Manders, D. B., Morón, A., McIntire, D., Miller, D. S., Richardson, D. L., Kehoe, S. M., Albuquerque, K. V., & Lea, J. S. (2018). Locally advanced cervical cancer: Outcomes with variable adherence to treatment. *American Journal of Clinical Oncology, 41*(5), 447–451.

Martin, M. Y., Keys, W., Person, S. D., Kim, Y., Ashford, R. S. II, Kohler, C., & Norton, P. (2005). Enhancing patient-physician communication: A community and culturally based approach. *Journal of Cancer Education, 20*(3), 150–154.

Masi, C. M., & Gehlert, S. (2009). Perceptions of breast cancer treatment among African American women and men: Implications for interventions. *Journal of General Internal Medicine, 24*(3), 408–414.

McDaniel, J. S., Musselman, D. L., Porter, M. R., Reed, D. A., & Nemeroff, C. B. (1995). Depression in patients with cancer: Diagnosis, biology, and treatment. *Archives of General Psychiatry, 52*, 89–99.

McDonald, P. A., Thorne, D. D., Pearson, J. C., & Adams-Campbell, L. L. (1999, Winter), Perceptions and knowledge of breast cancer among African-American women residing in public housing. *Ethnicity & Disease, 9*(1), 81–93.

Meichenbaum, D., & Turk, D. C. (1987). *Facilitating treatment adherence.* Plenum Press.

Meyerowitz, B. E., Formenti, S. C., Ell, K. O., & Leedham, B. (2000). Depression among Latina cervical cancer patients. *Journal of Social and Clinical Psychology, 19*(3), 352–371.

Miles, M. B., & Huberman, A. M. (1994). *Qualitative data analysis: An expanded sourcebook* (2nd ed.). Sage Publications.

Miller, S. M., Tagai, E. K., Wen, K.-Y., Lee, M., Hui, S.-kuen A., Kurtz, D., Scarpato, J., & Hernandez, E. (2017). Predictors of adherence to follow-up recommendations after an abnormal Pap smear among underserved inner-city women. *Patient Education and Counseling, 100*, 1353–1359.

Misra-Herbert, A. D. (2017). Cervical cancer in African American women: Optimizing prevention to reduce disparities. *Cleveland Clinic Journal of Medicine, 84*(10), 795–796.

Mitchell, J., Lannin, D. R., Mathews, H. F., & Swanson, M. S. (2002). Religious beliefs and breast cancer screening. *Journal of Women's Health, 11*(10), 907–915.

Mocciaro, F., Di Mitri, R., Russo, G., Leone, S., & Quercia, V. (2014). Motivational interviewing in inflammatory bowel disease patients: A useful tool for outpatient counselling. *Digestive and Liver Disease, 46*(10), 893–897.

Morgan, P. D., Barnett, K., Perdue, B., Fogel, J., Underwood, S. M., Gaskins, M., & Brown-Davis, C. (2006, January/ February). African American women with breast cancer and their spouses' perception of care received from physicians. *Association of Black Nursing Faculty Journal, 17*(1), 32–37.

Morgan, P., Fogel, J., Rose, L., Barnett, K., Mock, V., Davis, B. L., Gaskins, M., & Brown-Davis, C. (2005). African American couples merging strengths to successfully cope with breast cancer. *Oncology Nursing Forum, 32*(5), 979–987.

Morgan, P. D., & Gaston-Johansson, F. (2006). Spiritual well-being, religious coping, and the quality of life of African American breast cancer treatment: A pilot study. *Association of Black Nursing Faculty Journal, 17*(2), 73–77.

Naar-King, S., Outlaw, A., Green-Jones, M., Wright, K., & Parsons, J. T. (2009). Motivational interviewing by peer outreach workers: A pilot randomized clinical trial to retain adolescents and young adults in HIV care. *AIDS Care, 21*(7), 868–873. doi:10.1080/09540120802612824

NIH: National Cancer Institute. (2019). Cancer disparities. https://www.cancer.gov/about-cancer/understanding/disparities

Nonzee, N. J., Ragas, D. M., Ha Luu, T., Phisuthikul, A. M., Tom, L., Dong, X. Q., & Simon, M. A. (2015). Delays in cancer care among low-income minorities despite access. *Journal of Women's Health, 24*(6), 506–514.

Paladino, A. J., Anderson, J. N., Graff, J. C., Krukowski, R. A., Blue, R., Jones, T. N., Buzaglo, J., Kocak, M., Vidal, G. A., & Graetz, I. (2019). A qualitative exploration of race-based differences in social support needs of diverse women with breast cancer on adjuvant therapy. *Psycho-Oncology, 28*(3), 570–576.

Pascal, J., Hendren, S., Fiscella, K., Loader, S., Rousseau, S., Schwartzbauer, B., Sanders, M., Carroll, J., & Epstein, R. (2011). Understanding the processes of patient navigation to reduce disparities in cancer care: Perspectives of trained navigators from the field. *Journal of Cancer Education, 26*(1), 111–120.

Pasick, R. J., & Burke, N. J. (2008). A critical review of theory in breast cancer screening promotion across cultures. *Annual Review of Public Health, 29*, 351–368.

Paterniti, D. A., Melnikow, J., Nuovo, J., Henderson, S., DeGregorio, M., Kuppermann, M., & Nease, R. (2005). "I'm going to die of something anyway": Women's perceptions of tamoxifen for breast cancer risk reduction. *Ethnicity & Disease, 15*(3), 365–372.

Patton, M. Q. (2002). *Qualitative research and evaluation methods* (3rd ed.). Sage Publications.

Pullen, E., Perry, B., & Oser, C. (2014). African American women's preventative care usage: The role of social support and racial experiences and attitudes. *Sociology of Health & Illness, 36*(7), 1037–1053.

Reece, M. (2003). HIV-related mental health care: Factors influencing dropout among low-income, HIV positive individuals. *AIDS Care, 15*(5), 707–716.

Richardson, J. L., & Sanchez, K. (1998). Compliance with cancer treatment. In J. C. Holland (Ed.), *Psycho-oncology.* Oxford University Press, 67–77.

Richardson Gibson, L. M., & Parker, V. (2003, September/October). Inner resources as predictors of psychological well-being in middle-income African American breast cancer survivors. *Cancer Control, 10*(5), 52–59.

Robinson-White, S., Conroy, B., Slavish, K. H., & Rosenzweig, M. (2010). Patient navigation in breast cancer: A systematic review. *Cancer Nursing, 33*(2), 127–140.

Rongkavilit, C., Naar-King, S., Wang, B., Panthong, A., Bunupuradah, T., Parsons, J., . . . Phanuphak, S., Koken, J. A., Saengcharnchai, P., & Phanuphak, P. (2013). Motivational interviewing targeting risk behaviors for youth living with HIV in Thailand. *AIDS And Behavior*, *17*(6), 2063–2074. doi:10.1007/s10461-013-0407-2

Sadler, G. R., Ko, C. M., Cohn, J. A., White, M., Weldon, R., & Wu, P. (2007). Breast cancer knowledge, attitudes, and screening behaviors among African American women: The Black cosmetologists promoting health program. *BMC Public Health*, *7*(1), 57–64.

Sanders, K., Whited, A., & Martino, S. (2013). Motivational interviewing for patients with chronic kidney disease. *Seminars in Dialysis*, *26*(2), 175–179. doi:10.1111/sdi.12052

Sarr, M., Simoes, E. J., Murayi, T., Figgs, L. T., & Brownson, R. C. (1998). Trends in breast cancer screening in Missouri from 1987–1995, and predictions for the years 2000 and 2010. *Missouri Medicine*, *95*(12), 663–669.

Schraufnagel, T. J., Wagner, A. W., Miranda, J., & Roy-Byrne, P. P. (2006). Treating minority patients with depression and anxiety: What does the evidence tell us? *General Hospital Psychiatry*, *28*, 27–36.

Schubart, J. R., Farnan, M. A., & Kass, R. B. (2015). Breast cancer surgery decision-making and African-American women. *Journal of Cancer Education*, *30*(3), 497–502.

Selove, R., Kilbourne, B., Fadden, M. K., Sanderson, M., Foster, M., Offodile, R., Husaini, B., Mouton, C., & Levine, R. S. (2016). Time from screening mammography to biopsy and from biopsy to breast cancer treatment among black and white, women Medicare beneficiaries not participating in a health maintenance organization. *Women's Health Issues*, *26*(6), 642–647.

Sharma, M. (2012). Reinforcement-based treatment for alcohol and drug addictions. *Journal of Alcohol and Drug Education*, *56*(1), 86–88.

Shen, Y., Dong, W., Esteva, F. J., Kau, S-W., Theriault, R. L., & Bevers, T. B. (2007). Are there racial differences in breast cancer treatments and clinical outcomes for women treated at M.D. Anderson Cancer Center? *Breast Cancer Research & Treatment*, *102*, 347–356.

Sheppard, V. B., Walker, R., Phillips, W., Hudson, V., Xu, H., Cabling, M. L., He, J., Sutton, A. L., & Hamilton, J. (2018). Spirituality in African-American breast cancer patients: Implications for clinical and psychosocial care. *Journal of Religion and Health*, *57*(5), 1918–1930.

Sher, I., McGinn, L., Sirey, J. A., & Meyers, B. (2005). Effects of caregivers' perceived stigma and causal beliefs on patients' adherence to antidepressant treatment. *Psychiatric Services*, *56*, 564–569.

Smith, A., Vidal, G., Pritchard, E., Blue, R., Martin, M., Rice, L. S., Brown, G., & Starlard-Davenport, A. (2018). Sistas Taking a Stand for Breast Cancer Research (STAR) study: A community-based participatory genetic research study to enhance participation and breast cancer equity among African American women in Memphis, TN. *International Journal of Environmental Research and Public Health*, *15*(12), 1–12.

Smith-Bindman, R., Miglioretti, D. L., Lurle, N., Abraham, L., Ballard Barbash, R., Strzelczyk, J., Dignan, M., Barlow, W., Beasley, C., Kerlikowske, K. (2006). Does utilization of screening mammography explain racial and ethnic differences in breast cancer? *Annals of Internal Medicine*, *144*(8), 541–553.

Stelger, G., Samkoff, J., & Karoullas, J. (2003, Winter). A program of interventions designed to increase mammography rates in women ages 50 years and older for an underserved racial minority. *Journal of Health & Human Services Administration*, *26*(3), 336–349.

Steinberg, M. L., Fremont, A., Khan, D. C., Huang, D., Knapp, H., Karaman, D., Forge, N., Andre, K., Chaiken, L. M., & Streeter, O. E. (2006). Lay patient navigator program implementation for equal access to cancer care and clinical trials. *Cancer*, *107*(11), 2669–2677.

Strauss, A. L., & Corbin, J. (1990). *Basics of qualitative research: Grounded theory procedures and techniques*. Sage Publications.

Swenson, K. K., Nissen, M., & Henly, S. J. (2010). Physical activity in women receiving chemotherapy for breast cancer: Adherence to a walking intervention. *Oncology Nursing Forum, 37*(3), 321–330. doi:10.1188/10.ONF.321-330

Talley, C. H., Yang, L., & Williams, K. P. (2017). Breast cancer screening paved with good intentions: Application of the information-motivation-behavioral skills model to racial/ethnic minority women. *Journal of Immigrant and Minority Health, 19*(6), 1362–1371.

Taylor, K. L., Lamdan, R. M., Siegel, J. E., Shelby, R., Moran-Klimi, K., & Hrywna, M. (2003). Psychological adjustment among African American breast cancer patients: One-year follow-up results of a randomized psychoeducational group intervention. *Health Psychology, 22*(3), 316–323.

Tejeda, S., Darnell, J. S., Cho, Y. I., Stolley, M. R., Markossian, T. W., & Calhoun, E. A. (2013). Patient barriers to follow-up care for breast and cervical cancer abnormalities. *Journal of Women's Health, 22*(6), 507–517.

Thompson, D. R., Chair, S. Y., Chan, S. W., Astin, F., Davidson, P. M., & Ski, C. F. (2011). Motivational interviewing: A useful approach to improving cardiovascular health? *Journal of Clinical Nursing, 20*(9/10), 1236–1244. doi:10.1111/j.1365 2702.2010.03558.x

Ukachi, M. (2013). Motivational interviewing: Evidence-based strategy in the treatment of alcohol and drug addiction. *Psychologia, 21*(3S), 174–196.

Van Nes, M., & Sawatzky, J. V. (2010). Improving cardiovascular health with motivational interviewing: A nurse practitioner perspective. *Journal of the American Academy of Nurse Practitioners, 22*(12), 654–660. doi:10.1111/j.1745-7599.2010.00561.x

Wallner, L. P., Li, Y., McLeod, M. C., Hamilton, A. S., Ward, K. C., Veenstra, C. M., An, L. C., Janz, N. K., Katz, S. J., & Hawley, S. T. (2017). Decision-support networks of women newly diagnosed with breast cancer. *Cancer, 123*(20), 3895–3903.

Warren-Findlow, J., & Prohaska, T. R. (2008). Families, social support, and self-care among older African-American women with chronic illness. *American Journal of Health Promotion, 22*(5), 342–349.

Wells, A. A., Gulbas, L., Sanders Thompson, V., Shon, E., & Kreuter, M. W. (2014). African-American breast cancer survivors participating in a breast cancer support group: Translating research into practice. *Journal of Cancer Education, 29*(4), 619–25.

Wells, A., & Zebrack, B. (2008). Psychosocial barriers contributing to the under-representation of racial/ethnic minorities in cancer clinical trials. *Social Work in Health Care, 46*(2), 1–14.

Whyte, L. W. (2000). Promoting health prevention programs and medical compliance: An expanded conceptual model. In S. L. Logan & E. M. Freeman (Eds.), *Health care in the black community*. Haworth Press, 83–95.

Williams, D. (1992). A systematic approach for using qualitative methods in primary prevention research. *Medical Anthropology, 4*(4), 391–409.

Williams, K. P., Mullan, P. B., & Fletcher, F. (2007). Working with African American women to develop a cancer literacy assessment tool. *Journal of Cancer Education, 22*(4), 241–244.

Wilmoth, M. C., & Sanders, L. D. (2001). Accept me for myself: African American women's issues after breast cancer. *Oncology Nursing Forum, 28*(5), 875–879.

Wolf, R. L., Zybert, P., Brouse, C. H., Neugut, A. I., Shea, S., Gibson, G., Lantigua, R. A., & Basch, C. E. (2001). Knowledge, beliefs, and barriers relevant to colorectal cancer screening in an urban population: A pilot study. *Family and Community Health, 24*(3), 34–47.

Yan, A. F., Stevens, P., Holt, C., Walker, A., Ng, A., McManus, P., Basen-Enguist, K., Weinhardt, L. S., Underwood, S. M., Asan, O., & Wang, M. Q. (2017). Culture, identity, strength and spirituality: A qualitative study to understand experiences of African American women breast cancer survivors and recommendations for intervention development. *European Journal of Cancer Care, 28*(3), 1–15.

Module 2.2: Survivorship Care Plans

This module highlights the increased use of survivorship care plans (SCPs), an important development in cancer care. Just preparing these plans is insufficient, though; to be of value to low-income women of color, the plans must be shared with the patient and the primary care provider. Patients and families should have an opportunity to discuss and problem solve any troubling aspects of the plan before making the transition away from oncology care. In addition, navigators should take into account socioeconomic and cultural barriers to care, as well as resources for medical care and financial and emotional support that are available in the community. Strategies and resources to achieve "warm hand-offs," as the patient's care transitions to healthcare providers in the community, should be explored and included in the SCP. We conclude this module with an example of an SCP that been modified to include cultural and socio-ecological areas of relevance for low-income women of color.

Cancer Survivors

Survivorship is an important goal of efforts to decrease health disparities. Chronic care includes not only acute care but also continued management to ensure survivorship. Cancer survivorship begins with a diagnosis and continues throughout the individual's life. Survivors include not only individuals diagnosed with cancer but also others in their life, including family members and friends. With a growing number of individuals diagnosed with cancer who survive—approximately 16.9 million (National Cancer Institute, "Statistics") in the United States alone—it is important to address not only acute treatment but also long-term care for these individuals. Five-year relative survival statistics indicate that African American women have lower survival rates than White men and women and Black men and men and women of other racial/ethnic groups (Table 2.2). Studies indicate that cancer survivors commonly report issues with access to quality care, difficulty understanding and following treatment instructions, and a lack of resources to help manage comorbid illness following treatment (Institute of Medicine [IOM], 2006; National Research Council).

Table 2.2 Five-Year Relative Cancer Survival (%) by Race and Sex

	Male	Female
White	65.9	66.6
Black	63.1	58.0
Other	60.8	69.2

Cancer Survivorship Care Plans

A 2006 IOM report shared findings from research that examined the care received by cancer survivors. The data indicated that little guidance had been available for cancer survivors and/or their primary care providers to address the medical and psychosocial problems they were experiencing after treatment. To address the needs of the growing population of cancer survivors, the IOM (2006) recommended that survivors be provided with a summary of their treatments and a follow-up care plan (the SCP). It was also expected that the SCPs would be shared with primary care providers to ensure high-quality, guidelines-based care following cancer treatment.

The SCP represents an individualized summary of the effects that a survivor might experience based on her particular cancer diagnosis, the treatments that are/were recommended and completed, possible symptoms, and how symptoms might be prevented and/or treated (IOM, 2006). The SCP is also intended to include recommendations for the appropriate cancer screening regimen for the survivor, as well as a discussion of psychosocial (emotional, social, and legal) and financial issues that might arise as a result of the woman's cancer diagnosis and treatment. The SCP may include schedules for physical examination and medical tests to see if the cancer has spread to other parts of the body or if the cancer has returned following a cancer-free period. Follow-up care helps to detect health problems that may exist or arise, irrespective of the cancer diagnosis. The SCP also provides recommendations for a healthy lifestyle, such as consumption of fruits and vegetables, weight management, exercise, and quitting smoking, to improve cancer outcomes and overall health and quality of life. The SCP would ideally include referrals to specialists, including those capable of assisting with depression, anxiety, pain management, and so forth, as well as information about resources for support. Needless to say, this is a comprehensive and complicated document to complete.

In response to the 2006 IOM report and recommendation, many groups developed SCPs to help improve the quality of care and life of survivors as they completed cancer treatment. Despite efforts to follow the recommendation, scientific information to inform the content and expected outcomes of SCPs was scant, or plans were not responsive to minority survivors. However, the development and adoption of SCPs has spurred the development of templates for development and research related to their use and impact.

Early studies suggested inconsistent use of SCPs, despite requirements to do so (Guy et al., 2015; Yabroff et al., 2016). In a 2013 survey of employees of cancer programs across the United States who were knowledgeable about SCP use, most respondents reported that requirements prompted the use of SCPs, but 56% of respondents indicated that the plans were not used (Birken et al., 2013). The programs that reported SCP use indicated that they were used with breast and colorectal cancer survivors (Birken et al., 2013). More noteworthy, these plans were seldom reaching the survivors or their primary care providers. Respondents also reported on barriers to SCP use, including insufficient resources to complete the plans, perceived difficulty using them, and lack of advocacy for plan use. SCPs were more likely to be used in academic cancer centers and the National Cancer Institute's Community Cancer Centers (Birken et al., 2013).

A 2014 review of 42 studies further illustrated the limited information available to support the implementation of SCPs (Mayer et al., 2014). The studies suggested that although used only sporadically, SCPs were associated with improved patient knowledge about issues and concerns related to their care, and both survivors and providers were found to endorse their use (Mayer et al., 2014). Only four of the studies were randomized controlled trials, which avoid many biases associated with observational studies. Other limitations included cross-sectional or pre/post designs, limited generalizability due to lack of sample diversity, and lack of systematic testing of data-collection tools. A survey of oncology clinical staff suggested that the time needed to obtain information and complete the plans was a barrier to their use. Although patients reported that the plans were useful, primary care physicians reported insufficient knowledge of cancer survivorship issues and concerns to implement them (Dulko et al., 2013). These findings raise issues related to institutional support, in terms of both time and training, for the implementation of SCPs.

Another recent criticism of SCPs is that they have shown little evidence of improving health outcomes and healthcare delivery, particularly for more distal health outcomes (Jacobsen et al., 2018). A systematic review of 13 randomized studies found that SCPs generally did not improve the most commonly assessed outcomes of physical, functional, and psychological well-being. However, the authors concluded that it is premature to say that SCPs are not beneficial, given weaknesses in the evidence base such as a limited number of studies, heterogeneity in their content and delivery, and unrealistic expectations that administering it only once would improve patient outcomes weeks or months later (Jacobsen et al., 2018). Despite these negative findings, the authors did report more positive proximal outcomes (e.g., information received and improved care delivery), particularly when the SCP is accompanied by counseling to prepare survivors for future clinical encounters (Jacobsen et al., 2018). For example, patient navigators can use SCPs to coach survivors in how to raise concerns about their survivorship issues at subsequent visits with providers. The navigator should update the SCP with the survivor, ensure the survivor's physician receives a similarly updated version, and provide brief education on survivorship issues (Jacobsen et al., 2018).

More recent research has increased confidence in the use of SCPs and identified areas to consider as they are implemented. A scoping review sought to determine how primary care physicians have been involved in SCP use and the extent to which these plans have been effective in improving survivor cancer care (LaGrandeur et al., 2018). The 25 studies identified as relevant to the review suggested that SCPs increased the confidence of primary care providers in managing the care of survivors and increased the survivors' quality of life and well-being. The studies suggested that it is important to determine the best delivery mode to increase the usefulness of SCPs for patients and providers (LaGrandeur et al., 2018). A secondary data analysis of the 2014 The Behavioral Risk Factor Surveillance System (BRFSS) cancer survivorship module (1,855 cancer survivors) was performed to determine whether SCPs were associated with health behaviors believed to be correlated with long-term outcomes for cancer survivors (Shay et al., 2019). The study found that receiving an SCP was associated with having a recent medical appointment (important to follow-up screening and care), exercise in the past month, non-smoking status, and up-to-date mammography, which are all important lifestyle issues for cancer survivors. SCPs were not associated with colorectal cancer screening, and only 37% of those surveyed reported receiving a SCP (Shay et al., 2019), suggesting the need to ease the burden of preparing and delivering these plans.

Given the increasing evidence of the value of SCPs for cancer patients' outcomes, they have received continued endorsement. The American Society for Clinical Oncology (ASCO) endorses their use and has developed a template that supports development of the treatment summary and a follow-up care plan to enhance communication and coordination of care. ASCO has developed SCP templates for breast cancer, colorectal cancer, non-small cell and small cell lung cancer, prostate cancer, and diffuse large B-cell lymphoma cancer (ASCO, "Survivorship Care Planning Tools"). The National Cancer Institute ("Follow-up Medical Care"), American Cancer Society (ACS, "Survivorship Care Plans"), and the Centers for Disease Control and Prevention (CDC, "Cancer Survivorship Care Plans") provide information on cancer survivorship and the use of SCPs. The ACS also provides links to cancer survivorship templates (ACS, "Survivorship Care Plans"), while the CDC has developed and published "A National Action Plan for Cancer Survivorship." OncoLife has developed a template that cancer survivors can use to develop an SCP ("Cancer Survivorship Care Plan").

However, Ashing-Giwa et al. (2013) found that SCPs need to be modified to increase their usability for minorities and developed an SCP template that includes cultural and socio-ecological modifications. Based on their Community-Based Participatory Research, CBPR adapted SCPs 'were found' to be more responsive to African American breast cancer survivors and to increase their applicability and acceptability among diverse ethnic minority cancer survivor populations.

Racial and ethnic differences in the survivorship experience may be present, but again there is limited information on this issue. More research is needed to fully understand variations in cancer outcomes. One study found that only a small number of participants reported receiving SCPs; those who did not receive an SCP reported a greater number of health information needs (Kent et al., 2013). Low-income and minority patients are more likely to experience financial hardship following a cancer diagnosis compared to other patients (Yabroff et al., 2016), and there is a need to understand how financial hardship affects risk for poor cancer outcomes. Cancer treatment is expensive and difficult to manage for those without health insurance, for those with incomes below the poverty level, and for older adults who do not yet qualify for Medicare (Guy et al., 2015). Studies have identified decreased and discontinued hormonal therapy adherence among breast cancer survivors and delays in receipt of medical care and prescription renewals (Burg et al., 2015; Hershman et al., 2015; Kent et al., 2013).

African Americans and Native American women have high rates of obesity, which may influence cancer outcomes (White et al., 2014). Obesity may be associated with racial and ethnic differences in adverse cancer treatment experiences, such as lymphedema and cancer-related fatigue (Schmitz et al., 2014). African American and Native American cancer survivors may need assistance with weight management, dietary changes, and physical activity.

The role of social stressors, such as poverty and exposure to violence, has also been discussed with respect to disparities in cancer outcomes. These exposures are hypothesized to alter the neuroendocrine stress response and influence tumor biology and cancer outcomes (Volden & Conzen, 2013).

Thus, it is important to ensure that all of these issues are taken into account and more detailed information is provided to assist these patients and ensure the SCP's utility. Patients will also need help discovering accessible, acceptable resources and support, as well as obtaining support and assistance in implementing complex recommendations.

Some SCPs are specific to healthcare providers and should be completed and/or reviewed by these professionals. However, there are roles for other professionals. These include (1) ensuring that both the patient and her designated primary care provider receive the plan, (2) providing support during plan review, and (3) performing periodic reviews to determine adherence and reduce nonadherence to plan components. Social workers and patient navigators, including peer navigators and/or community health workers, may also facilitate the completion of these complicated documents. SCPs have utility to the extent that they provide reasonable and practical information, as well as supports to implement plan elements. Social workers, health educators, and peer and lay community health workers may play an important role in identifying these services and assisting patients as they seek to secure services to address health care, basic needs, referrals for psychological needs and concerns, as well as social support. Box 2.1 describes elements that might be completed by these staff.

Box 2.1 The Roles of Patient Navigators and Community Health Workers in Cancer Survivorship

Identification of Services and Resources for Inclusion

Assess and ensure inclusion of community-based resources to meet basic needs.

Assess and ensure inclusion of resources to assist with the costs of health and healthcare, including treatments and medication.

Identify and ensure inclusion of community-based health and healthcare resources with the capacity to meet cultural and linguistic needs.

Identify and ensure inclusion of culturally and linguistically appropriate education materials and information.

Identify and ensure inclusion of community-based, culturally and linguistically appropriate resources for social support.

Assess need for and ensure inclusion of spiritual support resources.

Identify and ensure inclusion of community-based, culturally and linguistically appropriate resources to assist with personal care.

Assistance and Linkage

Assist patients, families, and caregivers to overcome health system barriers.

Facilitate timely access to healthcare, including preventive care and future screening and detection protocols, as well as psychosocial care.

Link survivors to tobacco cessation, diet, and physical activity services.

Link survivors to behavioral health resources and spiritual resources as requested.

Link survivors to chronic disease self-management tools.

Provide patients, families, and caregivers with health education information and materials.

Link survivors to educational, vocational, and career support services.

Support

Review cancer survival care plan with patient and family; facilitate questions to providers; consider health literacy and comprehension.

Monitor, discuss, and problem solve adherence to cancer survival care plan.

Support survivors' efforts to make changes in their lifestyle and activities.

Support survivors' use of behavioral health resources, including support groups.

Support survivors' chronic disease self-management activities.

Discuss and address ongoing health information needs of patient, family, and caregivers.

Support family and caregivers with identification of support and respite care as needed.

A patient's quality of life following a cancer diagnosis is tied to her ability to manage her treatment and follow-up care. Self-management is a component of chronic care management. By providing key skills and knowledge, chronic care management is designed to offer methods for patients to feel prepared to play an active role in the management of their care and health (Barlow et al., 2008). Today's successful self-management programs build on the chronic disease self-management model developed by Lorig and Barlow (Barlow et al., 2008).

Adapted SCP

The following SCP is modified based on cultural and socio-ecological areas of relevance. Updated items or revisions made to the SCP are indicated by **_bolded, italicized text_**, while original elements of the plan are indicated in plain text.

What Is an SCP?
- A survivorship care plan (SCP) is an individualized summary and follow-up of your cancer treatment history and ideas for staying healthy.
- It helps you and your healthcare provider understand one another.
- A plan to keep with your healthcare records and to share with your primary care provider.

Why Is an SCP Important?
- The Institute of Medicine (IOM) researched the state of care for cancer survivors and found that little guidance is available for cancer survivors and their healthcare providers to overcome the medical and psychosocial problems that may arise post-treatment.

How Can I Use an SCP?
- It is meant for you to review and discuss with your healthcare team (both oncology and primary care).
- It should say when you need to get follow-up tests and which healthcare providers are responsible for your care.
- Bring it with you whenever you go to the doctor.
- Keep your SCP and refer to it so you can be sure you get the care and resources you need.
- It is very important to review your SCP with your cancer care team.

What Information Do I Need to Create an SCP?
- You may need to talk to your cancer care team to have some details of your cancer therapy available:
  1. Type of cancer
  2. If you underwent surgery, what procedures were done?
  3. If you received chemotherapy, what medications were received?
  4. If you received radiation therapy, what type of cancer was this done for?

General Information
- Patient name
- Date of birth

- Patient phone
- Patient email
- *Sex assigned at birth (male, female, other, decline to answer)*
- *Current gender identity (male, female, transgender male/transman/FTM, transgender female/transwoman/MTF, gender queer, additional category [please specify])*
- *Race/ethnicity*
- *Religious affiliation*
- Age at diagnosis
- Current age
- *Employment status (employed, unemployed, fulltime, parttime)*
- *Financial status (stable, strained, etc.)*

Healthcare Providers (Name/Institution)
- Primary care provider
- Surgeon
- Radiation oncologist
- Medical oncologist
- Other providers (*e.g., patient navigator, social worker, nurse practitioner, nutritionist*)

Treatment Summary
Diagnosis
- Cancer type/location subtype (*e.g., breast, colorectal, cervical*)
- Diagnosis date (*month*/year)
- Stage (I, II, III, *IV*, not applicable)
- *Metastatic sites (if applicable)*
- *TNM status (if applicable) (TNM stands for "tumor, node, metastasis," a system used to describe the spread and amount of cancer in the body. T describes the size of the tumor; N describes the spread of the cancer to nearby lymph nodes; M describes metastasis, or the spread of cancer to body parts other than the original site. TNM staging is used to describe most cancer types.)*
- Recurrences

Treatment
- Surgery (yes/no)
  - Surgery date(s) (*month*/year)
  - Surgical procedure/location (e.g., lumpectomy, hysterectomy)
- Radiation (yes/no)
  - Dose
  - Body area treated
  - End date (*month*/year)
- Immunotherapy (yes/no)
  - *Names of medication used*
  - Start dates (*month*/year)
  - End dates (*month*/year)
- Persistent symptoms or side effects at completion of treatment (no/yes/type[s])

Familial Cancer Risk Assessment
- Genetic (related to genes/heredity; passed from parents to children) risk factor(s) or predisposing conditions

- Genetic counseling (yes/no)
- Genetic testing results

Follow-up Care Plan
- Need for ongoing adjuvant (drug/method to enhance effectiveness of cancer treatment) treatment (yes/no)
- Additional treatment name
- Planned duration
- Possible side effects

Schedule of Clinical Visits
- Coordinating provider
- When? How often?

Cancer Surveillance or Other Recommended Related Tests
- Coordinating provider
- What? When? How often?
- Please continue to see your primary care provider for all general healthcare recommended, including cancer screening. Any symptoms should be brought to the attention of your provider, including (1) anything that represents a brand-new symptom; (2) anything that represents a persistent symptom; and (3) anything you are worried about that might be related to the cancer coming back.
- Possible late- and long-term effects that someone with this type of cancer and treatment may experience
- *Comorbid diagnoses (e.g., high blood pressure, diabetes, obesity, asthma) (pre-cancer and post-cancer)*
- Possible effects on treatment
- *Side effects (undesirable effects of a drug or medical treatment): sexual concerns (e.g., vaginal dryness, painful intercourse, decreased desire); osteoporosis or osteopenia; cardiomyopathy; cardiac arrhythmia (abnormal heartbeat); left ventricular dysfunction or heart failure; infertility; acute myeloid leukemia (AML) or myelodysplasia (MDS); persistent numbness, tingling in hands and/or feet; cognitive changes (memory loss; difficulty with short-term memory, concentration, or learning new skills); fatigue (overwhelming physical, mental, or emotional exhaustion); other (please indicate)*

Psychosocial Concerns (new section)
- Cancer survivors may experience issues with the areas listed below. If you have any concerns in these or other areas, please speak with your doctors or nurses to find out how you can get help with them.
  - Emotional/mental health
  - Physical functioning
  - Memory or concentration loss
  - Fatigue
  - Insurance
  - Parenting
  - Weight changes
  - School/work
  - Fertility

- Stopping smoking
- Finances
- Sexual functioning
- Other
- *Financial concerns*
  - High cost of cancer care
  - Lost job/inability to find work
  - Insurance co-pays
  - No insurance
  - Loss of ability to work
  - Transportation costs
  - Loss of partner's income (due to taking time off from work for caregiving)
  - Losing employer-based insurance
  - Other
- *Consequences of financial concerns/burdens*
  - Borrowing money
  - Going into debt
  - Filing for bankruptcy
  - Making financial sacrifices
  - Worrying about paying large medical bills
  - Inability to cover costs of medical care
  - Loss of partner's income (due to taking time off from work for caregiving)
  - Other

Resources You May Be Interested In (new section)

- *American Institute for Cancer Research*
- *Cancer Financial Assistance Coalition*
- *Cancer and Careers*
- *Cancer Support Community*
- *CancerCare*
- *Job Accommodation Network*
- *Journey Forward*
- *LIVESTRONG*
- *LIVESTRONG Survivorship Centers of Excellence*
- *National Coalition for Cancer Survivorship*
- *National Cancer Survivors Day Foundation*
- *OncoLife Survivorship Care Plan*
- *National Cancer Institute: Office of Cancer Survivorship*
- *National Coalition for Cancer Survivorship*
- *Patient Advocate Foundation*
- *Save My Fertility*
- *Healthcare Hospitality Network*
- *ACS Hope Lodge Program*
- *Mercy Medical Angels*
- *ACS Road to Recovery Program*
- *Meals on Wheels*
- *United Way 211*
- *Assist Fund*
- *Patient Advocate Foundation*
- *African American Breast Cancer Alliance (AABCA)*
- *Latinas Contra Cancer*
- *National LGBT Cancer Network*
- *National LGBT Cancer Project*
- *Sisters Network Inc.*
- *Black Women's Health Imperative*
- *National Asian Women's Health Organization (NAWHO)*
- *Circle of Life*
- *Other*

Additional Commentary
- *Your personal experiences*
- *Your questions*
- *Advance care plans (Advance care planning involves making decisions about what care you want to receive at a time when you may not be able to speak for yourself. This decision-making process includes you, your family, your loved ones, and your healthcare providers. The goal is to maintain and maximize your independence as you prepare for the end of life.)*
- *Durable power of attorney (Durable power of attorney authorizes someone to handle matters, like finance or healthcare. They are legal documents created in advance planning and remain in effect if you become mentally incapacitated or unable to handle your own affairs.)*
- Other comments
- Prepared by (name)
- Delivered on (date)

References

American Cancer Society. Survivorship care plans. https://www.cancer.org/treatment/survivorship-during-and-after-treatment/survivorship-care-plans.html

American Society for Clinical Oncology. Survivorship care planning tools. https://www.cancer.org/treatment/survivorship-during-and-after-treatment/survivorship-care-plans.html

Ashing-Giwa, K., Tapp, C., Brown, S., Fulcher, G., Smith, J., Mitchell, E., Santifer, R. H., McDowell, K., Martin, V., Betts-Turner, B., Carter, D., Rosales, M., & Jackson, P. A. (2013). Are survivorship care plans responsive to African American breast cancer survivors? Voices of survivors and advocates. *Journal of Cancer Survivorship, 7,* 283–291.

Barlow, J., Wright, C., Sheasby, J., Turner, A., & Hainsworth, J. (2008). Self-management approaches for people with chronic conditions: A review. *Patient Education and Counseling, 48,* 177–187.

Birken, S. A., Mayer, D. K., & Weiner, B. J. (2013). Survivorship care plans: prevalence and barriers to use. *Journal of Cancer Education, 28*(2), 290–296.

Burg, M. A., Adorno, G., Lopez, E. D., Loerzel, V., Stein, K., Wallace, C., & Sharma, D. K. (2015). Current unmet needs of cancer survivors: analysis of open-ended responses to the American Cancer Society Study of Cancer Survivors II. *Cancer, 121,* 623–630.

Centers for Disease Control and Prevention. Cancer survivorship care plans. https://www.cdc.gov/cancer/survivors/life-after-cancer/index.htm

Centers for Disease Control and Prevention (CDC). A national action plan for cancer survivorship: Advancing public health strategies. https://stacks.cdc.gov/view/cdc/6536/

Dulko, D., Pace, C. M., Dittus, K. L., Sprague, B. L., Pollack, L. A., Hawkins, N. A., & Geller, B. M. (2013). Barriers and facilitators to implementing cancer survivorship care plans. *Oncology Nursing Forum, 40*(6), 575–580.

Guy, G. P. Jr., Yabroff, K. R., Ekwueme, D. U., Virgo, K. S., Han, X., Banegas, M. P., Soni, A., Zheng, Z., Chawla, N., & Geiger, A. M. (2015). Healthcare expenditure burden among non-elderly cancer survivors, 2008–2012. *American Journal of Preventive Medicine, 49*, S489–S497.

Hershman, D. L., Tsui, J., Wright, J. D., Coromilas, E. J., Tsai, W. Y., & Neugut, A. I. (2015). Household net worth, racial disparities, and hormonal therapy adherence among women with early-stage breast cancer. *Journal of Clinical Oncology, 33*, 1053–1059.

Institute of Medicine. (2006). *From cancer patient to cancer survivor: Lost in transition.* National Academies Press. http://georgiacore.org/articleImages/articlePDF_396.pdf

Jacobsen, P. B., DeRosa, A. P., Henderson, T. O., Mayer, D. K., Moskowitz, C. S., Paskett, E. D., & Rowland, J. H. (2018). Systematic review of the impact of cancer survivorship care plans on health outcomes and health care delivery. *Journal of Clinical Oncology, 36*, 2088–2100. http://ascopubs.org/doi/full/10.1200/JCO.2018.77.7482

Kent, E. E., Forsythe, L. P., Yabroff, K. R., Weaver, K. E., de Moor, J. S., Rodriguez, J. L., & Rowland, J. H. (2013). Are survivors who report cancer-related financial problems more likely to forgo or delay medical care? *Cancer, 119*, 3710–3717.

LaGrandeur, W., Armin, J., Howe, C. L., & Ali-Akbarian, L. (2018). Survivorship care plan outcomes for primary care physicians, cancer survivors, and systems: A scoping review. *Journal of Cancer Survivorship, 12*(3), 334–347.

Mayer, D. K., Birken, S. A., Check, D. K., & Chen, R. C. (2014). Summing it up: An integrative review of studies of cancer survivorship care plans (2006-2013). *Cancer, 121*(7), 978–996.

National Cancer Institute. Follow-up medical care. https://www.cancer.gov/about-cancer/coping/survivorship/follow-up-care

National Cancer Institute, Office of Cancer Survivorship. Statistics. https://cancercontrol.cancer.gov/ocs/statistics/statistics.html

National Research Council. 2006. From Cancer Patient to Cancer Survivor: Lost in Transition. Washington, DC: The National Academies Press. https://doi.org/10.17226/11468

OncoLife. Cancer survivorship care plan. https://oncolife.oncolink.org/

Schmitz, K. H., Agurs-Collins, T., Neuhouse, M. L., et al. (2014). Impact of obesity, race and ethnicity on cancer survivorship. In D. J. Bowen, G. B. Denis, & N. A. Berger (Eds.), *Impact of energy balance on cancer disparities.* Springer, 63–90.

Shay, L. A., Schmidt, S., Dioun, S. I., Grimes, A., & Embry, L. (2019). Receipt of a survivorship care plan and self-reported health behaviors among cancer survivors. *Journal of Cancer Survivorship, 13*(2), 180–186.

Volden, P. A., & Conzen, S. D. (2013). The influence of glucocorticoid signaling on tumor progression. *Brain, Behavior, and Immunity, 30*, S26–S31.

White, M. C., Espey, D. K., Swan, J., Wiggins, C. L., Eheman, C., & Kaur, J. S. (2014). Disparities in cancer mortality and incidence among American Indians and Alaska Natives in the United States. *American Journal of Public Health, 104*, S377–S387.

Yabroff, K. R., Dowling, E. C., Guy, G. P., Banegas, M. P., Davidoff, A., Han, X., Virgo, K. S., McNeel, T. S., Chawla, N., Blanch-Hartigan, D., Kent, E. E., Li, C., Rodriguez, J. L., de Moor, J. S., Zheng, Z., Jemal, A., & Ekwueme, D. U. (2016). Financial hardship associated with cancer in the United States: Findings from a population-based sample of adult cancer survivors. *Journal of Clinical Oncology, 34*, 259–267.

Module 2.3: Clinical Trial Uptake: Additional Options
for Treatment

This module discusses clinical trials, an option that sometimes broadens cancer treatment options. Clinical trials may represent a significant opportunity to improve cancer health equity among low-income women of color. In this module we discuss the problem of clinical trial underrepresentation among women and persons of color and the barriers to inclusion and participation. We conclude with story illustrations that feature four common scenarios that we might see in real-world practice, with possible interpersonal strategies to help encourage participation.

Absence of diverse populations in clinical trials is a barrier to effective implementation of interventions that can support effective care. Improving involvement of various populations in clinical trials is part of the work on making the expanded CCM more appropriately generalizable to other populations. One of the greatest potentials for reducing cancer mortality in high-risk populations is through increasing participation in cancer clinical trials. Cancer prevention and treatment clinical trials ultimately offer a high level of hope for reducing ethnic cancer disparities by increasing scientific knowledge (Polite et al., 2017). Without participation, we cannot learn whether findings apply equally or whether there are racial and ethnic differences in response to therapy (Kaplan, 1997). However, the disproportionate underrepresentation of ethnic minorities and women in cancer clinical trials funded by the National Cancer Institute (NCI) (U.S. Preventive Services Task Force, 2010) makes the potential for reducing the burden of cancer mortality in these high-risk populations a pressing challenge (Baum & Houghton, 1999; Christian & Trimble, 2003; Nazha et al., 2019). Despite significant national collaborative efforts (e.g., the 1993 NIH Revitalization Act, which encouraged proportional representation of women and minorities in research sponsored by the National Institutes of Health [Subtitle B: S131-133]), the problem of underrepresentation in cancer clinical trials is still a major barrier to reducing health disparities (Nazha et al., 2019). Although members of racial and ethnic minorities in the United States are at greater risk of dying from their cancer diagnosis (National Institute of Health, 2002), they are also less likely to participate in cancer clinical trials (Nazha et al., 2019; U.S. Preventive Services Task Force, 2010). Although many of the same challenges related to clinical trial participation exist for heart disease (e.g., hypertension), there seems to be more stigma associated with a cancer diagnosis (National Cancer Institute, 2002), especially when we consider the disproportionately low rates of minority participation in trials. Thus, it is important to emphasize elements of cultural relevance associated with cancer prevention and treatment trial participation because many of the barriers to participation occur within a sociocultural context that impacts patients' beliefs and attitudes (Graham et al., 2016; Wells & Zebrack, 2008).

Underrepresentation by Specific Subgroups

Unfortunately, only 2% to 5% of all adult cancer patients in America participate in clinical trials (Comis et al., 2003; Du et al., 2009; Ford et al., 2007; Melisko et al., 2005; Sateren et al., 2002), and rates are even lower for minority populations. Relative to White patients, lower enrollment rates were noted in African Americans, Hispanics, and Asian/ Pacific Islanders (Steward, 2007). And when four types of cancer (breast, colorectal, lung, and prostate) were considered in aggregate, Hispanics and African Americans were underrepresented in cancer clinical trials (Murthy et al., 2004). This is particularly alarming given the higher rates of cancer mortality among minorities.

The problem of clinical trial underrepresentation is also documented among women (Del Carmen & Rice, 2015; Duma et al., 2018; Killien et al., 2004; Mishkin et al., 2016; Murthy et al., 2004). Despite the importance of diversity of cancer trial participants, there is also little attention given to the lack of women in such trials, particularly high-impact studies of non–sex-specific cancers (Jagsi et al., 2009). However, Jagsi et al. (2009) found that studies that received government funding support included a higher proportion of female participants. Whether the rationale for including minorities and women is framed in terms of equity in access to clinical trials, generalizability of the results, or the need for valid subgroup analyses, participation over the past two decades has fallen short of the mark.

There are several important consequences of this underrepresentation in terms of science and health disparities. Although ethnic minority groups have been included in experimental studies for many years, the actual number of participants is so disproportionately small that meaningful statistically significant analysis cannot be performed (Advani et al., 2003; Brawley & Freeman, 1999; Brown & Topcu, 2003; Buring, 2000; Corbie-Smith et al., 1999; Hoel et al., 2009; Moreno-John et al., 2004; Murthy et al., 2004; Pierce et al., 2003; Sateren et al., 2002; Yancey et al., 2005). To date, the majority of clinical trials have included a somewhat limited portion of the U.S. population: middle-class, married white males (Schmotzer, 2012; Swanson & Ward, 1995). Evidence indicates that certain groups, such as women and ethnic minorities (Janson, 2001; Schmotzer, 2012), the elderly (Brown & Topcu, 2003; Lang & Lidder, 2010; Moreno-John et al., 2004), and the poor are underrepresented in clinical research (Erves et al., 2017; NIH/NCI, 2002), and this lack of participation is often due to barriers (Ahluwalia et al., 2002). Despite national collaborative efforts among government agencies, professional organizations, and patient advocates, the problem of underrepresentation of ethnic minorities is still a major barrier to reducing health disparities.

Given the alarming cancer mortality rates and the valuable data obtained from cancer treatment trials, it is imperative that ethnic minorities and women have the opportunity to participate in these trials (Linden et al., 2007). One of the greatest potentials for reducing cancer mortality in high-risk populations is through increasing participation in cancer clinical trials (Wells & Zebrack, 2008). Effective treatment methods and interventions for cancer and other diseases are dependent on clinical trial research (Lawsin et al., 2007). If trials do not include minorities, then it's unclear whether the results of the research are generalizable and relevant to everyone. A consequence of insufficient valid scientific findings from clinical trials is that data relevant to minority populations may not support adequate guidance to the best care for patients (Powell et al., 2008). For the results of a clinical trial to be clinically useful, the sample must be representative of the patient population (Kemeny et al., 2003). Underrepresentation in clinical trials leads to insufficient data and clinical practice recommendations.

Ultimately, the goal of clinical cancer research is to advance knowledge and improve decision-making in cancer care. Clinical trials focused on cancer prevention and treatment serve health professionals and the public by translating the insights of the biological and public health sciences into effective health interventions. The NCI provides support for the evaluation of cancer prevention and treatment strategies through clinical trials. According to the Institute of Medicine, improving opportunities for culturally sensitive recruitment and accrual of underrepresented populations to cancer clinical trials is a necessary step in addressing the public health impact of cancer health disparities.

Barriers to Clinical Trial Participation

Medically underserved populations, including low-income and racial/ethnic minority populations, face substantial barriers to receiving state-of-the-art cancer care throughout the continuum of cancer care, from preventive services to detection, treatment, and survival (Ford et al., 2007). Identifying both barriers and enablers becomes useful when we think about clinical trial uptake intervention targets, which should take a multilevel approach. The following barriers are well documented in the literature: (1) intrapersonal, (2) sociocultural, (3) interpersonal, (4) environmental, and (5) community/institutional (Table 2.3).

Intrapersonal Barriers
Psychological uncertainty and fear due to injections, needles, and pain have been documented as barriers to clinical trial participation. Patients report fear over "too much risk" in terms of personal safety and side effects (Du et al., 2009; Johnson et al., 2003). Others feel there is "no personal benefit to clinical trials" (Corbie-Smith et al., 1999; Pierce et al., 2003) and fail to see any need given their current good health. Some may not perceive research to be of critical, immediate, or priority interest in their communities (Norton & Manson, 1996).

Table 2.3 Clinical Trial Barriers and Enablers

	Intrapersonal	Sociocultural	Interpersonal	Environmental	Community/Institutional
Barriers	✓ Fear ✓ Personal risk/safety ✓ "No personal benefit"	✓ Cultural beliefs ✓ Family decision-making ✓ Alternative health practices ✓ Isolation ✓ Lack of trust ✓ Language barriers	✓ Lack of communication ✓ Disconnect with healthcare system ✓ Family/social commitments and conflicts	✓ Low socioeconomic status ✓ Practical/concrete barriers ✓ Access issues	✓ Lack of leadership ✓ Insufficient funding ✓ Health insurance reimbursement limits ✓ Minority underrepresentation
Enablers/Strategies	✓ Knowledge/awareness/understanding ✓ Increased discussion	✓ Education and relationship building with community	✓ Building trust with family and community ✓ Strengthening patient–provider relations	✓ Practical services and support (transportation, scheduling flexibility, etc.)	✓ Increased minority provider representation ✓ Improve funding ✓ Changes in policy

At this level, enablers and strategies should include improving patients' knowledge, awareness, and understanding (Brown & Topcu, 2003) and discussing the direct benefits of the trial and participation as an option. Educating the patient about the trial can help alleviate her psychological concerns by personalizing and prioritizing health.

Sociocultural Barriers

Minority populations can be mistrusting, suspicious, and skeptical about clinical trials and medical research and thus reluctant to participate (Alvidrez & Areán, 2002; Corbie-Smith et al., 1999; Freedland & Isaacs, 2004; Freedman, 1998; Hussain-Gambles et al., 2004; Moreno-John et al., 2004). They might wonder whether physicians would be fully honest with them about the risks and procedures, given historical injustices in research. This mistrust often spills over into the entire institution where physicians and researchers conduct clinical trial research (Ryan et al., 1998; Shavers et al., 2002). These feelings of isolation can affect health-related attitudes, beliefs, behaviors, and access to care. Other sociocultural influences include fatalistic beliefs about treatment and mortality, family decision-making, and the use of alternative health practices (Advani et al., 2003; Pierce et al., 2003; Swanson & Ward, 1995).

Enablers and strategies at this level should include working with communities to educate and empower trusted community ambassadors and trained laypersons who can educate people and encourage them to receive screening (Myers, 1999).

Interpersonal Barriers

Interpersonal barriers center around communication problems, such as a lack of understanding of informed consent (Corbie-Smith et al., 1999; Hussain-Gambles et al., 2004)—for instance, misunderstanding about guidelines; limited formal education or "hidden illiteracy" (Ahluwalia et al., 2002); and lack of information needed to evaluate whether participation is a viable option (Fouad et al., 2001; Sandler et al., 2001). Services and resources to overcome language and communication barriers are inadequate (Hussain-Gambles et al., 2004). For example, African Americans have been shown to feel disconnected and excluded from health decisions (King & Brunetta, 1999), and other minority groups feel that too much information or not enough guidance is provided (Jones et al., 2006); some report that they don't have an opportunity to ask questions or they feel rushed into making a decision. Other interpersonal barriers have been connected to social networks (Brown & Topcu, 2003; Fouad et al., 2001; Glanz et al., 2002) and family time commitments and/or conflict with family obligations (Fouad et al., 2001; Brown & Topcu, 2003).

Strategies to address these interpersonal barriers involve developing more trust by strengthening the therapeutic alliance between patients and providers (Corbie-Smith et al., 1999; Sandler et al., 2001). Trust encourages relationships and connections with individuals in hard-to-reach communities, which is necessary for minority enrollment in clinical trials. In addition, eliciting support from family members can promote participation (Pierce et al., 2003). Another factor that increases participation is knowing a health professional who is compassionate and competent or knowing a relative who has participated in a cancer clinical trial (Advani et al., 2003; Coyne et al., 2004; Pierce et al., 2003).

Environmental Barriers

Many practical barriers prevent minority populations from participating in cancer clinical trials, such as lack of transportation; lack of telephone, computer, or internet access; interference with work or job responsibilities; lack of time; inconvenience; complicated recordkeeping requirements; and difficulty rescheduling appointments due to the lack of flexibility on the part of study personnel (Advani et al., 2003;; Brown & Topcu, 2003; Chyun et al., 2003; Corbie-Smith et al., 1999; Coyne et al., 2004; Fouad et al., 2001; Freedland & Isaacs, 2004; Janson, 2001; Myers, 1999; Pierce et al., 2003; Robinson et al., 1996).

Strategies to address this problem can involve ensuring that participants have transportation to the study site, being flexible in scheduling appointments, and providing other practical services and support. These improvements often require increased funding.

Community/Institutional Barriers

Community and institutional barriers can often affect uptake to clinical trials. Such macro-level barriers include the lack of funding for institutional infrastructure supporting basic, clinical, psychosocial, and applications research programs (Eyre & Feldman, 1998). This lack of infrastructure can also involve insufficient leadership and partnerships between research institutions and community leaders. Health insurance companies are reluctant to reimburse providers for the costs associated with the delivery and administration of clinical trial protocols (Brown & Topcu, 2003), and this can create larger systems-level barriers. In addition, the number of minority academic cancer researchers is extremely small (Christian & Trimble, 2003), and this underrepresentation can affect clinical trial uptake because it can decrease the ability for an institution to build trust with underserved groups and minority individuals.

Many of the strategies used to address these problem will involve increased funding and development of policies and initiatives to broaden access to clinical trials (Murthy et al., 2004). Medical centers can improve minority representation in research by partnering with professional organizations, community leaders, advocacy organizations, and research institutions. For instance, holding a health fair can serve as a way to educate community members about clinical trial participation and to regain the community's trust (Cooper at al., 2002; Sateren et al., 2002). Finally, institutions should try to recruit clinicians and scholars from more diverse ethnic and minority populations. Better representation of women and persons of color on staff can promote trust in the institution by community members and lead to a more positive perception that the institution will be sensitive and knowledgeable about issues that concern them, their family, and their community.

Storyboard Illustrations

The following four storyboard scenarios illustrate common profiles of low-income women of color who face barriers to cancer prevention and treatment clinical trial participation. These scenarios can be used to identify an important individual in the women's support network who can help address barriers to enable and facilitate participation in clinical trial uptake.

Dialog 1

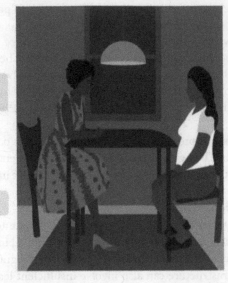

Mom, I overheard that you were recruited to be part of a cancer prevention trial due to our history of breast cancer.

Yeah...I was. But I'm not so sure I want to do it.

I think it's a good idea, Mom. You can find better ways to prevent diseases like breast cancer and other illnesses that we have in our family. This can help you and our family.

Hmmm. I'm still not sure.

Not only will you be able to find new ways to improve your health, but you can help other people in our family. Think about your grandbabies! And my grandbabies!

Well if it means taking care of my grandbabies, I'll consider it!

Clinical Trials Conversation: Mary (patient) and **Shiela** (daughter)
Setting: Family home
Barriers to Uptake: Minority underrepresentation, family decision-making, "no personal benefit"
Strategies: Including family in decision-making process and educating them on benefits

Dialog 2

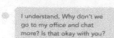

Based on your current condition, Mrs. Reyes, we recommend you start on this new cancer clinical trial. We think it will be very beneficial for your health. Our team will be with you every step of the way, for any of your concerns and questions. Please tell me your thoughts about this?

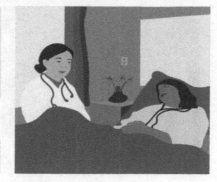

Dr. Cortez, with all respect, I've heard about these clinical trials and I don't really want to do it. I don't want to feel like a guinea pig and not be able to leave or stop the trial.

I understand. Why don't we go to my office and chat more? Is that okay with you?

Those are very legitimate fears. I understand where you are coming from.

The good thing is that these clinical trials are highly monitored and under extensive supervision, meaning that you will be taken care of throughout the process. And you can back out at any time.

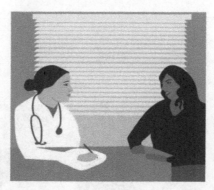

Yeah, but aren't there other risks, like side effects and longer treatment periods? My friends have warned me about that.

That's a good point. There are definitely some risks, but there are quite a few benefits as well, including having access to new research treatments before they are widely used as well as having expert advice and medical care throughout your journey. And your healthcare team will be with you through the entire experience. Here is some more information about the trial, and we can talk through it together with your family if you like.

Thank you for the information, Dr. Cortez. I will talk it over with my husband first and consider it.

Clinical Trials Conversation: Mrs. Reyes (patient) and **Dr. Cortez** (physician)
Setting: Observation room and private waiting room
Barriers to Uptake: Lack of communication and isolation
Strategies: Building trust and addressing personal safety

Dialog 3

Hello Ms. Jamila. My name is Anna and I am your Patient Navigator.

How do you feel about this clinical trial that your doctor spoke to you about?

I'm still just not sure what to expect. It's just really hard to think about all of this and know what to do.

That's a really legitimate question. We will be here to help you along the way if you have any questions.

After today we can help you schedule your first few visits. Before the first trial, we will work with you and the oncologist to make sure you are prepared for the first tests and make sure your family is aware as well, of everything.

Ok, but what happens from here?

Let's talk about this more in the clinic so I can show you some information!.

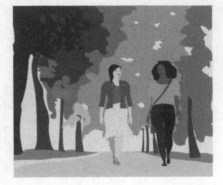

Following the first treatment, we will be there to help answer any of your questions about next steps. You will be given another appointment. You can call us at any time throughout the process. We want to make sure you are as comfortable as possible.

Thank you. That is helpful to know.

Can I have your telephone number to call you if I have questions?

Of course, here is my telephone number. Please call me at any time. That is what our team is here to do.

Ms. Jamila, is it ok if I call you next week to check in on you and answer any questions?

Sure. Thank you, Anna.

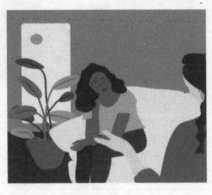

Clinical Trials Conversation: Ms. Jamila (patient) and **Anna** (patient navigator)
Setting: In community taking a walk and community clinic office
Barriers to Uptake: Lack of communication, lack of support
Strategies: Building trust and addressing behavioral skills

Dialog 4

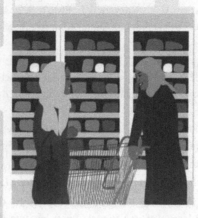

Hey Fatima! It's so good to see you! How have you been? I haven't seen you at the mosque lately.

Hey Mariam! I've been okay. My doctor recently recommended me to a clinical trial for my cancer treatment, but I'm not sure if I want to do it.

That's how we felt too before sending my mother through her clinical trial, but she was really well taken care of throughout the process. The doctors and team really made sure she was taken care of and that all her concerns were addressed. Our family was in the loop through the whole process.

And how did the doctors and nurses feel about your mom's hijab?

The team was very understanding and assigned her an all-female team to make sure she was comfortable.

That's great to know!

Of course. So good to see you, Fatima! Let us know if you need anything.

Clinical Trials Conversation: Fatima (patient) and **Mariam** (friend)
Setting: Local grocery store
Barriers to Uptake: Sociocultural issues, family decision-making, trust
Strategies: Education and communication

References

Advani, A. S., Atkeson, B., Brown, C. L., Peterson, B. L., Fish, L., Johnson, J. L., Gockerman, J. P., & Gautier, M. (2003). Barriers to the participation of African-American patients with cancer in clinical trials. *Cancer, 97*(6), 1499–1506.

Ahluwalia, J. S., Richter, K., Mayo, M. S., Ahluwalia, H. K., Choi, W. S., Schmelzle, K. H., & Resnicow, K. (2002). African American smokers interested and eligible for a smoking cessation clinical trial: Predictors of not returning for randomization. *Annuals of Epidemiology, 12*, 206–212.

Alvidrez, J., & Areán, P. (2002). Psychosocial treatment research with ethnic minority populations: Ethical considerations in conducting clinical trials. *Ethics & Behavior, 12*(1), 103–116.

Baum, M., & Houghton, J. (1999). Contribution of randomized controlled trials to understanding and management of early breast cancer. *British Medical Journal, 319*, 568–571.

Brawley, O. W., & Freeman, H. P. (1999). Race and outcomes: Is this the end of the beginning for minority health research? *Journal of the National Cancer Institute, 91*(22), 1908–1909.

Brown, D. R., & Topcu, M. (2003). Willingness to participate in clinical treatment research among older African Americans and Whites. *Gerontologist, 43*(1), 62–72.

Buring, J. E. (2000). Women in clinical trials—A portfolio for success. *New England Journal of Medicine, 343*(7), 505–506.

Christian, M. C., & Trimble, E. L. (2003). Increasing participation of physicians and patients from underrepresented racial and ethnic groups in national cancer institute-sponsored clinical trials. *Cancer Epidemiology, Biomarkers & Prevention, 12*, 277S–283S.

Chyun, D. A., Amend, A. M., Newlin, K., Langerman, S., & Melkus, G. D. (2003). Coronary heart disease prevention and lifestyle interventions. *Journal of Cardiovascular Nursing, 18*(4), 302–318.

Comis, R. L., Miller, J. D., Aldigé, C. R., Krebs, L., & Stoval, E. (2003). Public attitudes toward participation in cancer clinical trials. *Journal of Clinical Oncology, 21*(5), 830–835.

Cooper, L. A., Hill, M. N., & Powe, N. R. (2002). Designing and evaluating interventions to eliminate racial and ethnic disparities in health care. *Journal of General Internal Medicine, 17*, 477–486.

Corbie-Smith, G., Thomas, S. B., Williams, M. V., & Moody-Ayers, S. (1999). Attitudes and beliefs of African Americans toward participation in medical research. *Journal of General Internal Medicine, 14*, 537–546.

Coyne, C. A., Demian-Popescu, C., & Brown, P. (2004). Rural cancer patients' perspectives on clinical trials: A qualitative study. *Journal of Cancer Education, 19*, 165–169.

Del Carmen, M. G., & Rice, L. W. (2015). Underrepresentation of women in clinical trials: Why gynecologic oncologists are worried. *Obstetrics & Gynecology, 125*(3), 616–619.

Du, W., Mood, D., Gadgeel, S., & Simon, M. S. (2009). An educational video to increase clinical trials enrollment among breast cancer patients. *Breast Cancer Research and Treatment, 117*(2), 339–347. doi:10.1007/s10549-009-0311-7

Duma, N., Vera Aguilera, J., Paludo, J., Haddox, C. L., Gonzalez Velez, M., Wang, Y., Leventakos, K., Hubbard, J. M., Mansfield, A. S., Go, R. S., & Adjei, A. A. (2018). Representation of minorities and women in ONCOLOGY clinical Trials: Review of the past 14 years. *Journal of Oncology Practice, 14*(1).

Erves, J. C., Mayo-Gamble, T. L., Malin-Fair, A., Boyer, A., Joosten, Y., Vaughn, Y. C., Sherden, L., Luther, P., Miller, S., & Wilkins, C. H. (2017). Needs, priorities, and recommendations for engaging underrepresented populations in clinical research: A community perspective. *Journal of Community Health, 42*(3), 472–480. doi:10.1007/s10900-016-0279-2

Eyre, H. J., & Feldman, G. E. (1998). Status report on prostate cancer in African Americans: A national blueprint for action. *CA Cancer Journal for Clinicians, 48*(5), 315–319.

Ford, J. G., Howerton, M. W., Lai, G. Y., Gary, T. L., Bolen, S., Gibbons, M. C., Tilburt, J., Baffi, C., Tanpitukpongse, T. P., Wilson, R. F., Powe, N. R., & Bass, E. B. (2007). Barriers to recruiting underrepresented populations to cancer clinical trials: A systematic review. *Cancer, 112*(2), 228–242. doi:10.1002/cncr.23157

Fouad, M. N., Partridge, E., Wynn, T., Green, B. L., Kohler, C., & Nagy, S. (2001). Statewide Tuskegee alliance for clinical trials. *Cancer, 91*, 237–41.

Freedland, S. J., & Isaacs, W. B. (2004). Explaining racial differences in prostate cancer in the United States: Sociology or biology? *Prostate, 62(3)*, 243–252.

Freedman, T. G. (1998). "Why don't they come to Pike Street and ask us?" Black American women's health concerns. *Social Science in Medicine, 47*(7), 941–947.

Glantz, K., Rimer, B. K., & Lewis, F. M. (Eds.) (2002). *Health behavior and health education* (3rd ed.). Jossey-Bass.

Graham, P. W., Kim, M. M., Clinton-Sherrod, A. M., Yaros, A., Richmond, A. N., Jackson, M., & Corbie-Smith, G. (2016). What is the role of culture, diversity, and community engagement in transdisciplinary translational science?. *Translational Behavioral Medicine, 6*(1), 115–124. doi:10.1007/s13142-015- 0368-2

Hoel, A. W., Kayssi, A., Brahmanandam, S., Belkin, M., Conte, M. S., & Nguyen, L. L. (2009). Under- representation of women and ethnic minorities in vascular surgery randomized controlled trials. *Journal of Vascular Surgery, 50*(2), 349–354. doi:10.1016/j.jvs.2009.01.012

Hussain-Gambles, M., Atkin, K., & Leese, B. (2004). Why ethnic minority groups are underrepresented in clinical trials: A review of the literature. *Health and Social Care in the Community, 12*(5), 382–388.

Jagsi, R., Motomura, A. R., Amaranth, S., Jankovic, A., Sheets, N., & Ubel, P. A. (2009). Underrepresentation of women in high-impact published clinical cancer research. *Cancer, 115*, 3293–3301.

Janson, S. L. (2001). Attrition and retention of ethnically diverse subjects in a multicenter randomized controlled research trial. *Controlled Clinical Trials, 22*, 236S–243S.

Johnson, R. E., Williams, R. D., Nagy, M. C., & Fouad, M. N. (2003) Retention of under-served women in clinical trials: A focus group study. *Ethnic Disparities, 13*, 268–278.

Jones, J. M., Nyhof-Young, J., Moric, J., Friedman, A., Wells, W., & Catton, P. (2006). Identifying motivations and barriers to patient participation in clinical trials. *Journal of Cancer Education, 21*(416), 237–242.

Kaplan, D. (1997). Giving clinical trials a try. *Patient Care, 31*(12), 8(1).

Kemeny, M. M., Peterson, B. L., Kornblith, A. B., Wheeler, J., Levine, E., Bartlett, N., Fleming, G., & Cohen, H. J. (2003). Barriers to clinical trial participation by older women with breast cancer. *Journal of Clinical Oncology, 21(12)*, 2268–2275.

Killien, M., Bigby, J. A., Champion, V., Fernandez-Repollet, E., Jackson, R. D., Kagawa-Singer, M., Kidd, K., Naughton, M. J., & Prout, M. (2004). Involving minority and underrepresented women in clinical trials: The National Centers of Excellence in Women's Health. *Journal of Women's Health & Gender Based Medicine, 9*(10), 1061–1070.

King, T. E., & Brunetta, P. (1999). Editorial: Racial disparity in rates of surgery for lung cancer. *New England Journal of Medicine, 341*(16), 1231–1233.

Lang, K. J., & Lidder, S. (2010). Under-representation of the elderly in cancer clinical trials. *British Journal of Hospital Medicine, 71*(12), 678–681.

Lawsin, C. R., Borrayo, E. A., Edwards, R., & Belloso, C. (2007). Community readiness to promote Latinas' participation in breast cancer prevention clinical trials. *Health & Social Care in the Community, 15*(4), 369–378. http://dx.doi.org/10.1111/j.1365-2524.2007.00695.x

Linden, H. M., Reisch, L. M., Hart, A., Jr, Harrington, M. A., Nakano, C., Jackson, J. C., & Elmore, J. G. (2007). Attitudes toward participation in breast cancer randomized clinical trials in the African American community: A focus group study. *Cancer Nursing, 30*(4), 261–269. doi:10.1097/01.NCC.0000281732.02738.31

Melisko, M. E., Hassin, F., Metzroth, L., Moore, D. H., Brown, B., Patel, K., Rugo, H. S., & Tripathy, D. (2005). Patient and physician attitudes toward breast cancer clinical trials: Developing interventions based on understanding barriers. *Clinical Breast Cancer, 6*(1), 45–54.

Mishkin, G., Minasian, L. M., Kohn, E. C., Noone, A. M., & Temkin, S. M. (2016). The generalizability of NCI-sponsored clinical trials accrual among women with gynecologic malignancies. *Gynecologic Oncology, 143*(3), 611–616.

Moreno-John, G., Gachie, A., Fleming, C. M., Nápoles-Springer, A., Mutran, E., & Manson, S. M. (2004). Ethnic minority older adults participating in clinical research: Developing trust. *Journal of Aging and Health, 16*(5), 93S–123S. doi:10.1177/0898264304268151

Murthy, V. H., Krumholz, H. M., & Gross, C. P. (2004). Participation in cancer clinical trials: Race-, sex-, and age- based disparities. *Journal of the American Medical Association, 291*(22), 2720–2726.

Myers, R. E. (1999). African American men, prostate cancer early detection examination use, and informed decision-making. *Seminars in Oncology, 26*(4), 375–381.

National Institutes of Health/National Cancer Institute (NIH/NCI) (2002). Cancer clinical trials: The in-depth program (NIH Publication No. 02-5051).

Nazha, B., Manoj, M., Rebecca, P., & Owonikoko, T. F. (2019). Enrollment of racial minorities in clinical trials: Old problem assumes new urgency in the age of immunotherapy. *American Society of Clinical Oncology Educational Book, 39*, 3–10. doi/full/10.1200/EDBK_100021

Norton, I. M., & Manson, S. M. (1996). Research in American Indian and Alaska Native communities: Navigating the cultural universe of values and process. *Journal of Consulting and Clinical Psychology, 64*(5), 856–860.

Pierce, R., Chadiha, L. A., Vargas, A., & Mosley, M. (2003). Prostate cancer and psychosocial concerns in African American men: Literature synthesis and recommendations. *Health and Social Work, 28*(4), 302–311.

Polite, B. N., Adams-Campbell, L. L., Brawley, O. W., Bickell, N., Carethers, J. M., Flowers, C. R., Foti, M., Gomez, S. L., Griggs, J. J., Lathan, C. S., Li, C. I., Lichtenfeld, J. L., McCaskill-Stevens, W., & Paskett, E. D. (2017). Charting the future of cancer health disparities research: A position statement from the American Association for Cancer Research, the American Cancer Society, the American Society of Clinical Oncology, and the National Cancer Institute. *CA Cancer Journal for Clinicians, 67*(5), 353–361.

Powell, J. H., Fleming, Y., Walker-McGill, C. L., & Lenoir, M. (2008). The Project IMPACT experience to date: Increasing minority participation and awareness of clinical trials. *Journal of the National Medical Association, 100*(2), 178–187.

Robinson, S. B., Ashley, M., & Haynes, M. A. (1996). Attitudes of African-Americans regarding prostate cancer clinical trials. *Journal of Community Health, 21*(2), 77–87.

Ryan, D. H., Kennedy, B. M., Smith, L. L., Tucker, E. W., Melancon, L. E., Phillips, B. H., Lassale, C. C., & Bray, G. A. (1998). Successful strategies for recruiting African Americans to prevention trials. *Cancer, 83*(S8), 1833–1835.

Sandler, G. R., Freedman, T. G., Kadushin, G., & Rankin, E. D. (2001). A call to action: Patients' access to clinical trials. *Health & Social Work, 26*(3), 96–200.

Sateren, W. B., Trimble, E. L., Abrams, J., Brawley, O. K., Breen, N., Ford, L., McCabe, M. Kaplan, R., Smith, M., Ungerleider, R., & Christian, M. C. (2002). How sociodemographics, presence of oncology specialists, and hospital cancer programs affect accrual to cancer treatment trials. *Journal of Clinical Oncology, 20,* 2109–2117. doi:10.1200/JCO.2002.08.056

Schmotzer, G. L. (2012). Barriers and facilitators to participation of minorities in clinical trials. *Ethnicity & Disease, 22*(2), 226–230.

Shavers, V. L., Lynch, C. F., & Burmeister, L. F. (2002). Racial differences in factors that influence the willingness to participate in medical research studies. *Annals of Epidemiology, 12,* 248–256.

Stewart, J. H., Bertoni, A. G., Staten, J. L., Levine, E. A., & Gross, C. P. (2007). Participation in surgical oncology clinical trials: Gender-, race/ethnicity-, and age-based disparities. *Annals of Surgical Oncology, 14*(12), 3328–3334.

Swanson, M., & Ward, A. J. (1995). Recruiting minorities into clinical trials: Toward a participant-friendly system. *Journal of the National Cancer Institute, 87*(23), 1747–1759.

U.S. Department of Health and Human Services. (2000, November). *Healthy People 2010* (2nd ed.) (Volume 1, pp. 3–3 to 3–32). U.S. Government Printing Office.

U.S. Preventive Services Task Force. (2010). Screening for abdominal aortic aneurysm: recommendation statement. http://www.ahrq.gov/clinic/uspstf05/aaascr/aaars.htm

Wells, A., & Zebrack, B. (2008). Psychosocial barriers contributing to the under-representation of racial/ethnic minorities in cancer clinical trials. *Social Work in Health Care, 46*(2), 1–14.

Yancey, A. K., Ortega, A. N., & Kumanyika, S. K. (2005). Effective recruitment and retention of minority research participants. *Annual Reviews of Public Health, 27,* 9.1–9.28. doi:10.1146/annurev.publhealth.27.021405.102113

Chapter 2 Takeaways

- Cancer disparities among low-income women of color are best addressed using community partnerships, peer community health navigators or community health workers, and evidence-based clinical interventions.
- Traditional survivorship care plans need to be modified and adapted for low-income women of color to take into account sociocultural areas of relevance. These plans should include sociocultural demographic information, treatment summaries should be more specific, financial concerns should be addressed, a list of community resources should be provided, and additional information should be offered such as personal experiences, questions for providers, and end-of-life planning.
- One of the greatest potentials for reducing cancer mortality in high-risk populations is through increasing participation in cancer clinical trials; however, there is documented evidence that women and minorities are underrepresented in these trials. Given that many of the barriers to participation occur within a sociocultural context that affects women's beliefs and attitudes, social marketing and other educational strategies (e.g., storyboards, educational videos and print material) can be used to emphasize important and culturally relevant benefits associated with clinical trial participation.

3

Evaluation of Cancer Interventions and Programs

Healthcare provider: "Well, for me, because I work with so many chronically ill patients and this is kind of a subset of probably what you're looking at, they have so many appointments. I mean their life just consists of so many doctors' appointments. And I think as a healthcare system we need to do a better job of finding ways to decrease the number because we know that the more appointments that they have, the more likely they're going to miss."

Wells et al., 2019, p. 61

Chapter 3 examines the role that program evaluation and community engaged evaluation and education strategies play in promoting adherence to cancer interventions. We program evaluation and the role that it plays in determining when and how to modify intervention strategies for women of color. In addition, we highlight community engagement as a strategy for gaining information on the unique cancer needs, concerns, information, education and preferences of women of color. We highlight community based participatory research as a community engaged research strategy ideal for addressing women's needs, concerns and preferences to support culturally relevant and appropriate interventions.

Module 3.1: Outcomes and Assessing Intervention Efforts

The topic of evaluation of interventions is vast, complicated, and critically important not only in understanding the effectiveness of programs but also in shaping policies and even laws that impact the lives of those we hope to assist. This module will provide an overview of some of the critical issues in evaluating interventions in a variety of settings with a focus on cultural competence and equity—intentionally thinking about whether the outcomes of programs and initiatives differ for marginalized or underrepresented groups. Evaluation guides further development of the chronic care model (CCM) toward greater effectiveness with communities such as low-income women of color.

Health-related fields (e.g., public health, social work, medicine, nursing) recognize the need to identify the evidence of effectiveness for different policies and programs, translate that evidence into recommendations, and increase the extent to which that evidence

Cancer Navigation. Anjanette A. Wells, Vetta L. Sanders Thompson, Will Ross, Carol Camp Yeakey, and Sheri R. Notaro, Oxford University Press. © Oxford University Press 2022. DOI: 10.1093/med/9780190672867.003.0004

is used in public health practice. The Department of Health and Human Services (DHHS) has provided an overview of how evidence-based public health (EBPH) has developed to meet those needs (DHHS, 2010). The origins of EBPH can be traced back to the 1970s and 1980s, when the field of medicine began to address the fact that recommendations from expert panels often omitted relevant studies and failed to provide clear evidence of which aspects of healthcare interventions improved health outcomes (DHHS, 2010). Over time, evidence-based medicine evolved to examine which combination of specific services and medical conditions would lead to improved health outcomes in actual practice, and for which patients. EBPH involves the development, implementation, and evaluation of effective programs and policies in public health by applying principles of scientific reasoning, including systematic use of data and information systems and appropriate use of behavioral science theory and program planning models (Brownson et al., 2003). Evidence for the effectiveness of interventions has been used since the turn of the century to achieve some of the most important advances in public health (e.g., vaccination, motor vehicle and workplace safety, fluoridation of drinking water, and recognition of tobacco use as a health hazard).

Addressing population-based health problems takes place within a context of limited resources, including finances and practitioner expertise, specific environmental and organizational contexts, social norms, and political will. As all of these elements change over time, EBPH is not a fixed concept. Investing in an ineffective intervention may result in the loss of funding for a program that actually improves health or prevents disease. To reinforce this point, the Centers for Disease Control and Prevention (CDC) commonly requires applicants responding to Funding Opportunity Announcements to use evidence-based interventions.

Evidence for the effectiveness of interventions—such as programs, practices, or policies—can be used to provide a rationale for choosing a particular course of action or to justify the allocation of funding and other resources. There is demand for evidence at many levels: Practitioners use it for program planning and internal policies, local managers use it to decide which programs to support, and senior managers in government and healthcare organizations use it to set priorities and make policy and funding decisions. History has demonstrated the importance of focusing on evidence-based decision-making in the planning and delivery of health promotion interventions. For example, in the late 1980s, a new treatment for breast cancer involving high-dose chemotherapy with autologous bone marrow transplantation was rapidly disseminated prior to careful evaluation. Before subsequent studies concluded that the new treatment was ineffective and should not be used, more than 30,000 women who had already received the treatment died sooner and suffered more than they would have had they not received the treatment (DHHS, 2010). As another example, some screening tests have been shown to be medically unnecessary or even harmful to patients (Gibert, 2020). In public health practice, numerous cases have demonstrated the significant impact of evidence-based reviews on policy, funding, or programmatic decisions (DHHS, 2010). For example, a review of the impact of 16 state laws that prohibited driving with a blood alcohol concentration exceeding 0.08% found that after the law was implemented in these states, there was an average decrease of 7% in alcohol-related motor vehicle deaths (Community Guide, 2010).

As these examples have demonstrated, practitioners must ensure that "practice-based research" involves a rigorous examination of evidence that is defined and evaluated within a public health context. Public health evidence can take many forms but is often divided into three categories for the purpose of planning and making decisions (Lomas et al., 2005):

1. Scientific information that is independent of context and often assesses whether an intervention such as a specific technology (e.g., screening test) works in a controlled clinical trial
2. Social science evidence that is rigorous but also context based—for instance, a worksite program with many variables, including length and intensity of program, the background and demographics of the specific subgroups of employees, and perceived support from the employer (DHHS, 2010)
3. Anecdotal and locally based, taking into account key elements such as budget limitations and political considerations.

In practical terms, evidence can be conceptualized on a continuum from objective to subjective:

- Scientific literature in systematic reviews
- Scientific literature in one or more journal articles
- Public health surveillance data
- Program evaluations
- Clinical reports
- Case studies
- Qualitative data
- Community members
- Other stakeholders
- Media/marketing data
- Word of mouth
- Personal experience

When we discuss evidence, it is important to distinguish between the efficacy and the effectiveness of an intervention:

- *Efficacy trials* focus on measuring internal validity—the extent to which an intervention produces the expected result under ideal circumstances
- *Effectiveness trials* focus on measuring external validity—the degree to which the study's findings can be generalized to other subgroups and contexts (Gartlehner et al., 2006).

Now that we have established the importance of EBPH, it is also critical that practitioners understand that the purpose of evaluation is to demonstrate effectiveness, program improvements, and efficiencies and to identify gaps, assets, and resources to enhance program implementation. Equally important is the acknowledgment of the additional benefits of evaluation, which include an increased ability to identify successful activities, abilities, and programs that work; to monitor progress; and to make modifications and enhancements. However, although evaluation is crucial, it does not guarantee funding as political will, competing needs, and community preferences can exert a great deal of influence on the process.

EBPH occurs in a cyclical manner, with a continuous loop of interrelated processes (Figure 3.1). First, the problem at hand must be identified (e.g., cancer health disparities

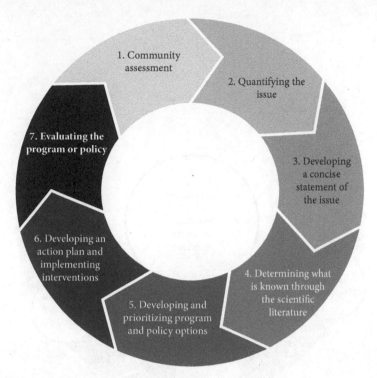

Figure 3.1 Cycle of evidence-based public health.

among low-income women of color). Next, a needs assessment or literature review should be conducted to understand the existing evidence as it relates to the particular targeted community. This assessment will help to focus the priority issues, ensuring a culturally appropriate approach, while further defining and identifying risk factors and barriers associated with the identified problem (e.g., lack of transportation for low-income women of color that prevents access to cancer screening). Next, an evidence-based approach or strategy known to have achieved success in the most cost-effective, reasonable manner should be selected (e.g., the CCM has been shown to promote cancer screenings, including mammography and Pap testing, in low-income African American women). The next step is to specify resources, activities, and anticipated outcomes (e.g., phone and print prompts designed to enhance Pap test compliance in women without hysterectomies), which then become key elements of the comprehensive evaluation plan.

CDC Model for Program Evaluation

The CDC has created an effective and useful six-step model for establishing a comprehensive program evaluation that provides examples of strategies for promoting cultural competence in each step (Figure 3.2). Informed by the American Evaluation Association's Public Statement on Cultural Competence in Evaluation, these strategies equip the practitioner with the tools to evaluate the program through a cultural competence lens (American Evaluation Association, 2014). The CDC (2014) stresses the importance of incorporating cultural competence into the evaluation process. Practitioners

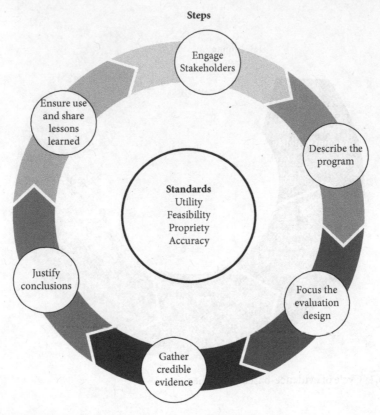

Steps

Figure 3.2   CDC framework for program evaluation.

should adapt approaches and methods to serve particular groups and communities with varied cultural backgrounds, worldviews, belief systems, strengths, and vulnerabilities. Planning and executing a culturally competent evaluation could reduce health disparities and improve health for all communities (CDC, 2014). Evaluators who choose to operate from a cultural competence lens purposely engage a range of stakeholders throughout the entire process to meet an ethical obligation of including everyone impacted by the evaluation.

Step 1: Engage the Stakeholders

While the CDC's model begins with engaging a diverse group of stakeholders, stakeholder engagement should be cultivated and maintained throughout the evaluation process. Indeed, practitioners must have a thorough understanding of all of the groups and individuals (e.g., patients, caretakers, physicians, administrators) who will be impacted by the intervention and/or have a substantive interest in the process or outcome. The key word here is "engagement," meaning that a process of consultation, listening, and sharing of information should be an integral component of planning and executing the evaluation. Many benefits accrue from stakeholder engagement, including providing credibility to the program and gaining assistance with the activities and overall implementation, advocacy, and sustainability.

To ensure that stakeholder engagement is undertaken in a culturally competent manner, practitioners must first take part in self-assessment and reflect on their personal background and life experiences that could influence how they conduct evaluations. This process of self-reflection exposes biases, prejudices, and assumptions we make about others, including those we serve. For instance, do you assume that other people share your worldview, values, and thought patterns? This might impede you from seeing community stakeholders as experts in their own right and could prevent you from engaging with "diverse segments of communities to include cultural and contextual dimensions important to evaluation" (American Evaluation Assessment, 2014). Culturally competent evaluators respect the cultures served in interventions by acknowledging that cultures and subcultures are varied and not static and that their own background (e.g., disciplinary training, race, ethnicity, socioeconomic status, religion, ideologies. language, sexual orientation, gender, gender identity) may place them in a privileged position with rights that others, including key stakeholders, cannot access.

Practitioners should take time to research the history of the community, potential distrust of prior interventions, and areas of disconnect between the evaluator and key stakeholders. To help build trust and establish a mutually beneficial working environment, practitioners may consider working with a co-evaluator or small advisory group from the community. These community members can then advise practitioners on expectations about meetings, communications, and procedures. Practitioners should also use their facilitation skills to monitor potential power imbalances among key stakeholders and to implement strategies to ensure equity among decision-makers, such as meeting separately with subgroups or soliciting some feedback anonymously (CDC, 2014).

Be sure to consider the language preference of key stakeholders in the evaluation process. To quote Nelson Mandela, former president of South Africa: "If you talk to a man in a language he understands, that goes to his head. If you talk to him in his language, that goes to his heart."

Step 2: Describe the Program

The next step is to describe the program's mission, vision, and goals in depth. Ensure that the program description reflects the diverse perspectives of the community. Several strategies are available to help with this stage of the evaluation:

1. Understand the stakeholders' perspectives of the program, as well as their priorities and worldview of illness and health. For example, some Eastern cultures consider disease and illness outside the control of the individual, a view that contrasts with a Western biomedical model (CDC, 2014). These different perspectives among stakeholders can then impact the perception of the program and the reception of the evaluation.
2. Consider ways in which race, politics, and privilege might impact the context of the evaluation.
3. Make sure the data that will be used to describe the community's needs are appropriate to the community; free of stigma, stereotypes, and externally assigned labels; and sensitive to within-group variation (CDC, 2014).

Careful crafting of "SMART" goals is a worthwhile effort to help ensure success of the program. SMART goals have several key components:

Specific (and strategic): Goals specify "who" and "what."
Measurable: Goals can be measured and specify "how."

Attainable: Goals are realistic and can be achieved in a specific amount of time.

Relevant (results oriented): The expected result is stated.

Timeframe: Goals have a clearly defined timeframe, including a target or deadline date.

For instance, the target of change might be low-income women of color, the desired change might be increases in cancer screening, and the timeframe might be at one year after the intervention.

The next component of describing the program is to create a logic model that details resources, activities, outputs, and outcomes (Figure 3.3). A logic model may result from a discussion with program staff and stakeholders, including participants. A linear or nonlinear logic model can serve as a graphical representation (e.g., boxes, arrow, drawings, pictures) of participants' stories and personal experiences that illustrate different perspectives, priorities, and foci.

Resources can also be thought of as inputs and can include staff (e.g., patient navigators), funds, research, equipment (e.g., mammography vans), facilities, and strengths and assets of the community. Activities may include training, education, outreach, vaccinations, and support groups. Outputs, which can be measured in several ways depending on the program, might include the number of people reached, the number of people served, or the number of people vaccinated. The outcomes measure the impact of the program over defined periods of time (e.g., short-term, intermediate, and long-term outcomes).

The CDC (2014) provides a relevant example of the ways in which the community can more accurately shape the description of the program in terms of the activities provided:

Evaluators of a heart disease program in a rural community interviewed community health workers (CHWs) to better understand whether home visits were implemented according to the procedure outlined in the CHW manual, were accomplished in the prescribed period, and received positive reactions from community members. The evaluators learned through their interviews that the primarily agrarian community responded more positively to home visits that exceeded the prescribed period of time.

CHWs explained the importance of taking as much time as needed to connect with community members. The evaluators understood the importance of having members of the community describe the program. Thus, when the evaluators presented their

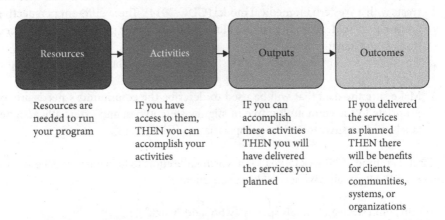

Figure 3.3 The logic model: a series of "if/then" statements.

results and recommendations, they included suggestions to modify the CHW manual to better reflect the needs of the community.

Step 3: Focus the Evaluation Design

After the logic model is conceptualized, the third step of the evaluation model is to work with stakeholders to focus the evaluation design. Evaluators should discuss the community's goals, values, definition of "success," and benefits to the community with the stakeholders to ensure their support, involvement, and shared understanding (CDC, 2014). Practitioners should choose evaluation questions that respect and reflect the community's perspectives and draw upon the knowledge gained during the first two steps of the evaluation process. Practitioners should seek to understand the community's information needs and plans for using the information that may not seem apparent or valuable to other people but are vitally important to them. The evaluation must also take into account the ways in which social, political, and cultural values influence an evaluation's design, implementation, and credibility within the community. Practitioners should explain evaluation design options and implications in terms that all stakeholders understand to account for differences in familiarity with formal evaluation and to help ensure that the findings are reliable and valid.

Some academic forms of evaluation (e.g., control groups) may seem unethical to some communities, who would prefer all members of the community to receive the intervention or program (CDC, 2014). Evaluators should discuss concepts of consent, confidentiality, participants' rights, data ownership, and data dissemination early in the evaluation process.

Step 4: Gather Credible Evidence

Stakeholders often have various values, opinions, and perspectives about what makes evidence legitimate or credible (e.g., quantitative data vs. process or qualitative data such as stories and photographs). Therefore, the evaluator should take care to solicit input from multiple stakeholders with the goal of taking into account stakeholder needs while ensuring that evaluation provides valid results within the context of the program (CDC, 2014). Data collection instruments should be culturally appropriate in light of the fact that most standardized instruments have been validated (found to be accurate) only with a dominant cultural group. Thus, any standardized instruments that are used must be tested for validity within the particular community. Practitioners must listen and respect the culture, ethnicity, language, political experience, age, class, gender, and other perspectives of stakeholders.

Several types of evaluation are typically employed throughout the research process:

- *Formative evaluations* identify issues and activities and monitor progress during program development.
- *Process evaluation* occurs during the program.
- *Summative evaluation* measures outcomes, effects, and changes in knowledge, skills, attitudes, and behaviors at the end of the program.

There are many quantitative and qualitative evaluation methods and tools (CDC, "Evaluation Documents"; Cottage Center for Population Health, "Cottage Health Evaluation Toolkit"; Indian Health Service, "Evaluation Toolkit"; Rural Health Information Hub, "Module 4") to help practitioners make sense of these three types of evaluations. Quantitative methods include questionnaires, surveys, pretests and post-tests, secondary data sources, and statistical analyses. Qualitative methods include interviews with key informants, focus groups, observations, and qualitative data analysis.

Planning the data collection design and methods requires the evaluator to consider the context and cultural characteristics of community members, as is the case with focus groups. Moderators should not make assumptions about participants or show preferences for particular experiences; rather, they should design and facilitate focus groups to ensure that all participants are comfortable speaking candidly and contributing with the least amount of conflict. In terms of observations of programs, stakeholders from the community can be enlisted to review the observation protocol, providing insight on cultural elements, practices, and norms that can inform the evaluation. The data collection plan should be mindful of additional cultural elements such as communication styles, nonverbal communication, the concept of time, possible need to match genders or ethnicities of interviewers and participants, power dynamics (including gatekeepers providing access to targets of interventions), and the importance of food and eating during sessions with interviewers or evaluators (CDC, 2014). The CDC (2014) provides a relevant vignette to illustrate the process of ensuring the cultural appropriateness of data collection instruments:

> An existing validated instrument was piloted as part of an evaluation that assessed risk factors related to heart disease and stroke. Some of the items in the instrument dealt with sensitive issues (e.g., cultural eating practices, cultural perceptions of attractive body images, cultural views on prescribed medications). Respondents were offended by some of the items, which they viewed as racial stereotypes. The inappropriate items led evaluators to conclude that participants would be reluctant or refuse to complete the evaluation protocol. Consequently, the evaluation team members discussed these issues, which resulted in a revised protocol for culturally appropriate communication and the subsequent revision of the data collection instrument.

Final considerations in the gathering of evidence include logistics, access to and availability of technology, and infrastructure, including the prevalence and reception of cellphones and availability of private space to conduct interviews.

At this point in the discussion of culturally appropriate evaluations, it is important to consider specific examples from prior interventions that have successfully incorporated equity into the evaluation strategy. Evaluations of programs should determine whether the program is differentially effective for certain populations or certain subgroups. For example, practitioners should guard against explicit and implicit biases that may operate in their evaluation of programs that target low-income populations; gender, ethnic, or sexual minorities; and/or other intersectional identities. To illustrate these challenges of evaluating programs through an equity lens, we provide an example from a federally sponsored employment program offered to low-income populations participating in the Temporary Assistance for Needy Families (TANF) program (Cavadel et al., 2018; Kautz et al., 2014).

The intervention's purpose was to enhance the self-regulation skills (e.g., ability to complete tasks, stay organized, and intentionally control emotions and behaviors) among a low-income sample of adults who participated in a coaching intervention for TANF recipients (Kautz & Moore, 2018). The evaluation team used an experimental research design to examine the effectiveness of coaching interventions that sought to help low-income individuals succeed in their jobs. The evaluation also examined the ef-ficacy of the implementation of the coaching interventions, the effectiveness or impact of coaching on self-regulation skills, and the role of self-regulation skills in generating any impacts on employment outcomes. The evaluation team posed three primary research questions:

1. What are the challenges of measuring self-regulation skills in the context of evalu-ations of employment programs that serve low-income populations?
2. What general criteria should evaluators use when selecting measures of self-regulation skills in this context?
3. What are the tradeoffs between different approaches for measuring self-regulation skills in this context?

Kautz and Moore (2018) discuss four challenges to measuring self-regulation skills in evaluations of employment programs for low-income populations. First, measures of self-regulation skills may reflect aspects of a person's background (e.g., socioeco-nomic status and financial status, race/ethnicity, education and literacy levels) in addi-tion to skills. Lower levels of literacy, for example, could impede the understanding of surveys designed to assess self-regulation skills. Second, most existing measures of self-regulation skills were developed to describe characteristics of populations generally or to diagnose severe problems, rather than to evaluate programs and interventions. Third, most existing measures were not designed for use or validated with low-income popula-tions. Fourth, some measures require too much time or special technology to administer.

Given these challenges, Kautz and Moore (2018) recommend that measures of self-regulation in the evaluation of employment programs should (1) relate to employment outcomes of interest; (2) capture skills that could be influenced by the program; (3) ac-count for confounding factors that affect measurement but not skills; and (4) be feasible to administer in an evaluation. To meet their criteria, they advocate for (1) using a set of general measures of self-regulation as well as ones that are specific to the employment context; (2) collecting information on other aspects of the participants' backgrounds that could be affected by the program; (3) modifying measures to fit the target pop-ulation; and (4) conducting analyses to assess the reliability and validity of selected measures.

Pretesting is a valuable tool that can help practitioners to modify measures so they better fit a particular population. In this example, a pretest was administered to a small group of people in the low-income target population in advance of the evaluation to en-sure that the literacy level of the surveys was appropriate. Based on follow-up in-depth interviews, one of the survey questions was modified to better explain the intent of the question.

Kautz and Moore (2018) recommend several analyses to test for reliability and va-lidity. Internal consistency or reliability measures the extent to which items designed to capture the same self-regulation skill are consistent with each other, as summarized with a statistic such as Cronbach's alpha. Measures with low reliability contain more measurement error, which may indicate that the measure fails to reflect the underlying skill. If the measures have too much measurement error, then the evaluation might not detect significant impacts in cases where the program does improve the under-lying skills (Kautz & Moore, 2018). Predictive validity is the correlation between meas-ures of self-regulation skills and employment outcomes: A high predictive validity indicates that the measures are linked to key outcomes. Discriminant validity is the extent to which measures designed to capture different self-regulation skills are statistically unrelated to each other, as measured by the correlation across conceptually different measures.

In summary, in their evaluation of self-regulation skills in a low-income population, Kautz and Moore (2018) present several ways to address the challenges that must be managed when conducting evaluations that focus on marginalized communities. The same principles applied in this example are useful when assessing patient navigation programs among low-income women of color. For example, practitioners could choose among a variety of both quantitative (e.g., questionnaires, pretests and posttests) and qualitative methods (e.g., key informant interviews, focus groups) to assess the outcomes of patient navigation such as changes in attitudes toward cancer screening and changes in adherence to medical appointments.

Justify Conclusions

The next step in the CDC (2014) evaluation model is to justify the conclusions that the practitioner has drawn by analyzing data, interpreting the findings, making judgments based on data, and making recommendations for using the findings. All stakeholders should be consulted in this critical phase of the evaluation to ensure that the evaluator's conclusions reflect the community's cultural values and perspectives. Because culture influences the definition, organization, classification, and interpretation of data, the evaluator must engage stakeholders during the data analysis phase. Because stakeholders may not be familiar with the components of data analysis, the evaluator should explain that data analysis entails organizing, classifying, tabulating, summarizing, comparing, and presenting the results of both qualitative and quantitative data in a manner that is easily understood.

Judgments about the program's effectiveness and worth are made by comparing the findings against other program outcomes and benchmarks, and these could differ for the stakeholders and the evaluators. Thus, the evaluator must understand the stakeholders' viewpoints and perspectives regarding the conclusions drawn from the data and attempt to reach a consensus on how to judge the program. Because not all judgments from an evaluation will be positive for all program stakeholders, the evaluator should discuss the implications that negative judgments might have on various stakeholders. Don't blame the program participants or the community; rather, focus on community strengths and opportunities for learning and growth.

To emphasize the importance of taking into consideration various cultural lens when interpreting data, the CDC (2014) provides a vignette to demonstrate the different conclusions that various stakeholders might draw from the same results:

In a recent evaluation of an asthma program, higher rates of emergency department visits for asthma were found among African-American children compared with their white counterparts. Some of the stakeholders interpreted this finding as a lack of motivation by the parents to schedule doctor appointments for appropriate asthma care and treatment. Stakeholders also believed that perhaps the finding suggested that the parents of the children with asthma did not prioritize health and preventive care. An alternate interpretation by other stakeholders was that this could be evidence that the health care system (e.g., policies, institutional factors) was failing to provide affordable insurance coverage for African-American children.

Ensure Use and Share Lessons Learned

The final step of the CDC (2014) model is to ensure that the findings are used and disseminated to maximize the lessons that are shared within the community and externally as well. Depending upon the context of the program, results of the intervention can be effectively disseminated in several ways, including townhall meetings, community forums, reports, peer-reviewed articles, and scientific conferences. To increase the likelihood that stakeholders will use and share the evaluation results, practitioners should facilitate an inclusive process to ensure that community members understand and value the results and recommendations of the evaluation and have an opportunity to discuss unintended consequences of the intervention. To increase buy-in and perceptions of legitimacy, the evaluator and community members may select a representative set of stakeholders who will be involved in establishing the evaluation's recommendations and envisioning a path to achieve and disseminate them.

When disseminating evaluation findings, practitioners should be flexible and willing to employ creative and varied presentation styles that may include photographs, drawings, and audiovisual elements. Alternatively, the community may be more receptive to hearing the findings from a key stakeholder who played an active role in the evaluation or on the advisory committee. It is prudent to pilot the presentation using focus groups, small group discussions, and individual meetings with those impacted by the evaluation's findings to assess their understanding of and reaction to particular presentation styles. The evaluation continues by working with stakeholders to develop concrete plans to use the information and implement recommendation to improve the community.

Concluding the Evaluation

To conclude the evaluation, practitioners should engage in a reflection period in which they examine the entire evaluation in the context of the community's unique culture and perspectives. Review evaluation results and recommendations with the stakeholders to assess both benefits and any unexpected harms that may have ensued. Take care to highlight the positive impact on the community and to promote future evaluations, while also working with community members to mitigate any negative effects. At the close of the evaluation, practitioners should ensure proper and thorough documentation of the procedures, decision-making process, lessons learned from community engagement, relationships that could be leveraged in future evaluations, and overall impact of adopting a cultural lens.

In addition to the CDC (2014) model of culturally competent evaluation, the Center for Culturally Responsive Evaluation and Assessment (CREA), located in the College of Education at the University of Illinois at Urbana-Champaign, is another resource for practitioners who seek to incorporate a cultural lens into the evaluation process (CREA, 2018). Based on an interdisciplinary model, CREA brings researchers together from multiple universities both domestically and internationally to design evaluations of social and educational interventions that acknowledge and respect the impact of cultural, cognitive, and interdisciplinary diversity.

CREA aims to integrate teaching, research, and scholarship relevant to both culturally sensitive and culturally responsive practices in evaluation and assessment in various fields, including education, social work, nursing, public health, and STEM-related disciplines. Culturally sensitive and responsive practices embrace culture as central to the research process. As Kofi Annan, former Secretary-General of the United Nations, said, "Intercultural dialogue, and respect for diversity are more essential than ever in a world where peoples are becoming more and more closely interconnected."

Summary

Practitioners who understand the importance of conducting culturally competent evaluations will take advantage of resources (e.g., CDC, 2014; CREA, 2018) that provide the concrete steps, skills, and theoretical evidence needed to ensure that evaluations are both effective and beneficial to a particular community. The practitioner's self-awareness of culture, biases, and worldviews is the critical first step toward conceptualizing an evaluation that will garner buy-in from the community, capitalize on their strengths, and mitigate their vulnerabilities. Engagement with stakeholders throughout the evaluation process is critical, especially during the stages of design, data collection, analysis, interpretation, recommendations, and dissemination of findings. Practitioners should remain vigilant and refresh their skills in cultural competence as they embark upon each new evaluation and new community, recognizing that their own backgrounds and life experiences may foster or hinder a successful evaluation that achieves the goals of improving health and well-being.

References

American Evaluation Association. (2014). Statement on cultural competence in evaluation. https://www.eval.org/Portals/0/Docs/aea.cultural.competence.statement.pdf

Brownson, R., Baker, E., Leet, T., & Gillespie, K. (2003). (Eds.) *Evidence-based public health.* Oxford University Press.

Cavadel, E., Kauff, J., Person, A., & Kravis, T. (2018). Perspectives on practice: A guide to measuring self-regulation and goal-related outcomes in employment programs. OPRE Report #2018-37. Office of Planning, Research, and Evaluation, Administration for Children and Families, U.S. Department of Health and Human Services. https://www.acf.hhs.gov/sites/default/files/documents/opre/50020_goals_measurebrief_final_508.pdf

Center for Culturally Responsive Evaluation and Assessment. (2018). https://crea.education.illinois.edu/home/about

Centers for Disease Control. Evaluation documents, workbooks and tools evaluation development tools. https://www.cdc.gov/eval/tools/developmenttools/index.html

Community Guide. (2010). From research to policy: lessons from a Community Guide review on alcohol-impaired driving laws. https://www.thecommunityguide.org/content/research-policy-lessons-community-guide-review-alcohol-impaired-driving-laws

Cottage Center for Population Health. Cottage health evaluation toolkit. https://www.cottage-health.org/population-health/learning-lab/toolkit/

Department of Health and Human Services. (2010). Evidence-based clinical and public health: Generating and applying the evidence. Secretary's Advisory Committee on National Health Promotion and Disease Prevention Objectives for 2020. https://www.healthypeople.gov/sites/default/files/EvidenceBasedClinicalPH2010.pdf

Gartlehner, G., Hansen, R., & Nissman, D. (2006). A simple and valid tool distinguished efficacy from effectiveness studies. *Journal of Clinical Epidemiology, 59,* 1040–1048.

Gilbert, N. (2020). The pros and cons of screening. *Nature, 579*(7800). https://doi.org/10.1038/d41586-020-00841-8

Indian Health Service. Evaluation toolkit. https://www.ihs.gov/sasp/training/evaluationtoolkit/

Kautz, T., Heckman, J., Diris, R., ter Weel, B., & Borghans, L. (2014). Fostering and measuring skills: Improving cognitive and non-cognitive skills to promote lifetime success. OECD Education Working Papers No. 110. https://doi.org/10.1787/5jxsr7vr78f7-en

Kautz, T., & Moore, Q. (2018). Measuring self-regulation skills in evaluations of employment programs for low-income populations: Challenges and recommendations. OPRE Report #2018-83. https://www.acf.hhs.gov/opre/report/measuring-self-regulation-skills-evaluations-employment-programs-low-income-populations

Lomas, J., Culyer, T., McCutcheon, C., McAuley, L., & Law, S. (2005). Conceptualizing and combining evidence for health system guidance. Canadian Health Services Research Foundation. https://www.cfhi-fcass.ca/migrated/pdf/insightAction/evidence_e.pdf

Rural Health Information Hub. Module 4: Evaluation tools for rural health promotion and disease prevention. https://www.ruralhealthinfo.org/toolkits/health-promotion/4/evaluation-tools

Wells, A., Thompson, V., Yeakey, C., Ross, W., & Notaro, S. (2019). *Poverty and Place: Cancer Prevention among Low Income Women of Color*. Plymouth, UK: Lexington Books, Inc.: Public Health Series.

Module 3.2: Community-Based Participatory Research

This module provides guidance on issues to consider when planning and designing community engagement efforts. It focuses on the beginning steps to forming a partnership, conducting a brief community needs assessment, and maintaining partnerships. Community-based participatory research (CBPR) offers a promising research methodology for arriving at the knowledge necessary to shape further developments in the chronic care model. Before we discuss some of the stages and logistics of the CBPR process from our work in Cincinnati, Ohio, we will define CBPR and a couple of basic terms associated with it (Israel et al., 2001). This module will conclude with a list of other terms often used in a discussion of CBPR.

What Is CBPR?

CBPR has emerged to bridge the gap between research and primary healthcare practice through community engagement and social action to increase health equity. Related names for CBPR include the following, which are all essentially "action research" approaches to addressing a particular problem or issue by partnering between researchers and the community:

- Community-engaged research (Israel et al., 1998; Reason & Rowan, 1981)
- Community-based participatory action research (Hills et al., 2007)
- Community-partnered participatory research (Jones, 2009)
- Community-based research (Centers for Disease Control and Prevention, 1997)
- Community participatory action (Jason et al., 2004)
- Participatory action research (Pyrch, 1991; Whyte, 1991)

- Citizen science (Irwin, 1995)
- Participatory health research (Fals-Borda & Rahman, 1991; International Collaboration for Participatory Health Research, 2013; Rifkin, 1996; Smithies & Webster, 1998)
- Participatory research (De Koning & Martin, 1996)

CBPR and related approaches involve more than community-placed research projects, which are projects that are based or placed in the community with its involvement but not full partnership (Israel et al., 1998). In contrast, CBPR and related approaches are systematic and intentional in terms of eliciting community members' expert knowledge and involvement in all phases of the research. Israel et al. (2001) defined CBPR as

> an applied collaborative approach that enables community residents to more actively participate in the full spectrum of research (from conception - design - conduct - analysis - interpretation - conclusions - communication of results) with a goal of influencing change in community health, systems, programs or policies. Community members and researchers partner to combine knowledge and action for social change to improve community health and often reduce health disparities.

This definition emphasizes that healthcare providers and key stakeholders are fully involved in each stage of research, as illustrated in Figure 3.4 (Tapp et al., 2013). This approach can also be used with interventions, education, and program development. It is often distinguished from other types of action research given the focus on public health.

The key principles of CBPR are as follows (Israel et al., 2001):

1. Recognizes community as a unit of identity
2. Builds on strengths and resources within the community
3. Facilitates collaborative, equitable involvement of all partners in all phases of the research
4. Integrates knowledge and action for mutual benefit of all partners
5. Promotes a co-learning and empowering process that attends to social inequalities
6. Involves a cyclical and iterative process
7. Addresses health from both positive and ecological perspectives
8. Disseminates findings and knowledge gained to all partners
9. Involves a long-term commitment by all partners.

What Is Community?

The definition of community (adopted by many researchers engaged in CBPR) is "those who have a shared unit of identity" (Burke et al., 2013). This definition is not limited to those who reside in a particular geographic area; rather, community is an expansive and inclusive concept and can include patients with shared health experiences (e.g., low-income women of color diagnosed with breast cancer or older African American women living with chronic diabetes) (Burke et al., 2013). A community can be diverse or homogeneous and can have differing sizes, socioeconomic backgrounds, and cultural

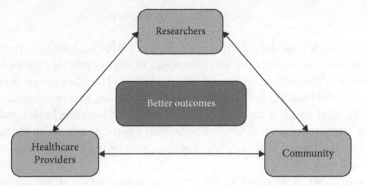

Figure 3.4 CBPR brings together researchers, healthcare providers, and community stakeholders to improve health outcomes.
(Tapp et al., 2013).

characteristics. In CBPR, identifying community is less about you as a researcher or practitioner identifying a static group of individuals with similar characteristics related to health and more about the process of asking questions and eliciting your own or a group's perception of community.

Who Is a Community Stakeholder?

CBPR has a long history of research based on relationships and partnerships with stakeholders. Stakeholders are people who are part of a community or the entire community, with a vested interest in an issue or problem. Similar to community, the term "stakeholder" has a somewhat diffuse definition that is based more on the process of asking questions about who is included in the process rather than a strict definition of who a stakeholder is "supposed to represent." The Agency for Healthcare Research and Quality (2017) refers to stakeholders as "persons or groups who have a vested interest in the clinical decision and the evidence that supports that decision" as well as "others who can bring insights on the patient perspective." This definition includes community members who have a "stake" in the issue or problem and/or have important information about the issue or problem.

When first identifying community stakeholders, it is important to ask "Are those who are most affected by the problem or have a stake in the issue at the table?" and "Do they carry key decision-making roles or have resources, knowledge, connections, or funding to address the problem or issue?" With consideration of who is impacted, this chapter will provide a range of examples of stakeholders (e.g., cancer survivors, family advocates, hair stylists well known in the community, community members, clinicians, church leaders and pastors) that can be considered when conducting CBPR. Although the process of identifying, engaging, and maintaining stakeholders in the research process can be daunting and overwhelming for many community-engaged researchers (Burke et al., 2013), it can also be an opportunity to form innovative and sustainable partnerships and to build trust and generate new ideas for communities in need.

Social Ecological Model

The social ecological model (SEM) is important to CBPR because it helps to explain other dimensions to individual-level influences and environmental choices to explain health behavior. This model considers that individuals and families are not isolated entities; they live and function in the context of neighborhoods and communities (Kumar et al., 2014). SEM entails a community understanding of health behavior and involves interdisciplinary approaches to interventions, with a particular focus on the social, cultural, and environmental factors influencing changes in an individual's behavior (Kumar et al., 2014; Stokols, 1996).

For example, when we consider adherence to mammogram screening for women of color who are at increased susceptibility for breast cancer, we must consider the context in which women live. Mammogram screening adherence goes beyond an individual woman's decision-making; there are multiple dimensions of influence on person–environment interactions. Although individual factors (like knowledge, attitudes, income, perceived health status) have an impact on whether a woman gets screening, it goes beyond that to involve other interpersonal factors (like family, friends, social support, marital status) as well as institutional and organizational influences (like church, school, organizational rules and policies). Community is made up of relationships established among institutions and organizations (like social networks and neighborhoods). SEM goes a step further and also considers the largest environmental spheres of public policy and systems (based on laws and policies at the local, state, and national level) (McLeroy et al.,1988). So while breast cancer mortality overall has been declining since the 1990s due to increases in awareness and early detection and treatment, women of color have not benefited equally. Thus, since factors that influence adherence and health behavior cannot be influenced by individual decisions alone, SEM provides an excellent framework for developing multidimensional solutions.

Phases in Conducting CBPR

Israel et al. developed seven core CBPR stages:

1. Forming a CBPR partnership
2. Assessing community strengths and dynamics
3. Identifying priority health concerns and research questions
4. Designing and conducting intervention and/or policy research
5. Feeding back in interpreting research findings
6. Disseminating and translating research findings
7. Maintaining, sustaining, and evaluating CBPR partnerships.

Though these phases follow somewhat of a sequential order, the process is actually more of a circular one (rather than linear), with some steps continuing throughout the entire CBPR effort (Israel, 2013; Israel et al., 2010). The following section includes a brief description of the CBPR stages, with examples from our research in Cincinnati, Ohio, and St. Louis, Missouri.

Pre-CBPR: Deciding Where to Focus Your Research Efforts

Before forming a CBPR partnership, we had to decide where to focus community health efforts. We began with the literature. We identified that Hamilton County, Ohio, is the most populous county in the tristate region (southwestern Ohio, northern Kentucky, southeastern Indiana) and home to its largest city. Incidence and mortality rates in Hamilton County and the United States as a whole support the extent of health disparities and cancer burden in this area. In Box 3.1, we feature some of these statistics and data. This information is critical to the development of targeted programs for cancer prevention, early detection, and control in Hamilton County and in similar densely populated U.S. cities. Social determinants that negatively affect cancer and health outcomes have deep historical roots in the legacy of segregation, resulting in high concentrations of poverty.

Box 3.1 Pre-CBPR: An Example of Where to Focus Your Research Efforts

---

With a population of 250,000 or more, Cincinnati is one of the most racially segregated cities in the United States. Compared to a U.S. poverty rate of 14% and an Ohio-wide rate of less than 15%, Cincinnati is also among the top 15 poorest cities in the country (CityLink Center, 2018). In Cincinnati we see the "ZIP code gap" reflected in the Community Needs Index (CNI) scores (Knudsen, 2017). CNI scores, ranging from 1 to 5 based on a high-level validated assessment, are an indicator for socioeconomic status variation, barriers to care, and increased need for healthcare services (Health Collaborative, 2016). A high CNI score is a warning sign that people living in this ZIP code are more likely to have difficulty accessing care, affording care, preventing and managing disease, obtaining an early diagnosis, having access to health information, and understanding medication and doctors' instructions (Health Collaborative, 2016).

For Hamilton County, the highest CNI score is 5 and the median CNI score is 3.7. Of the eight ZIP codes with the highest CNI in Cincinnati, six (those underlined below) will be included in the study sample recruitment. These Cincinnati neighborhoods are predominantly African American and have a higher-than-average population density, an extremely small number of families, and an extremely large number of single adults:

45203 (Queen City/West End), with a CNI score of 5
45214 (West End), with a CNI score of 5
45225 (Camp Washington), with a CNI score of 5
45232 (St. Bernard), with a CNI score of 5
45223 (Northside), with a CNI score of 4
45229 (Avondale), with a CNI score of 4.4
45219 (Corryville), with a CNI score of 4.4
45202 (Over-the-Rhine), with a CNI score of 4.4.

With a population of just over 800,000, Hamilton County and its diverse communities represent a multifaceted range of social determinants that can help answer the question of how place affects a community's health (Boeshart et al., 2015; Health Collaborative, 2016).

Phase 1: Forming a CBPR Partnership Through Engagement

This first stage involves identifying potential partners and communities to be involved in the research, building trust and relationships, establishing operating norms and CBPR principles to ensure equity and power sharing, and creating an infrastructure for carrying out the research process (Israel, 2013). This is the most important and fragile stage of CBPR. Community engagement is a viable strategy for addressing and examining health problems and needs in a community. It's impossible to advance to other stages without successfully completing this stage. The work done in this stage helps sustain the relationship through establishing and maintaining norms, continuing to build on trust and creating infrastructure for carrying out the research and future projects. A pitfall is for academics is to get too comfortable with the relationship and fail to obtain input from the community. This community engagement stage works best when there is a trusting, established relationship that is strengthened over time. Not even the most sophisticated, well-intentioned interventions will be successful if the stakeholders disagree with the approach. Box 3.2 provides an example of how to form a CBPR partnership through engagement.

Box 3.2 Phase 1: Forming a CBPR Partnership Through Engagement: An Example

Strategies to enhance cancer outreach, education, screening, and treatment should be based on input from not only target groups but also the community in which they live. Community members should also be allowed to voice their needs and shape solutions. Importantly, obtaining these perspectives first requires a *relationship*. We have built relationships with low-income communities of color, conducting community-engaged outreach to identify and partner with community partners and sites, as an entry for community connections and future community research and practice.

For one such engagement effort among the University of Cincinnati researchers and the local Cincinnati community, we spent one to two years identifying and engaging with community leaders and conducting relationship-building efforts. It took consistency and time to establish strong collaborative relationships through community outreach activities. We did a lot of the early legwork through quarterly delivery of "health baskets" with fruit, health education, and social service information (from local organizations like Planned Parenthood, American Cancer Society, National Alliance on Mental Illness, American Lung Association, United Way, and domestic violence shelters) for community members and stakeholders at the partnering churches, hair salons, and a social service agency, all in high-need Cincinnati neighborhoods. We also convened several luncheons and focus groups with community stakeholders (researchers, healthcare providers, church leaders and members, and hairstylists) in attendance. These luncheons were held on the university research campus as well as in the community at participating church sites. We used the luncheons as an opportunity not only to educate but also to receive input about critical needs, exploring the primary concerns related to the physical and mental health of the community.

Figure 3.5 illustrates community sites participating in community-engaged research.

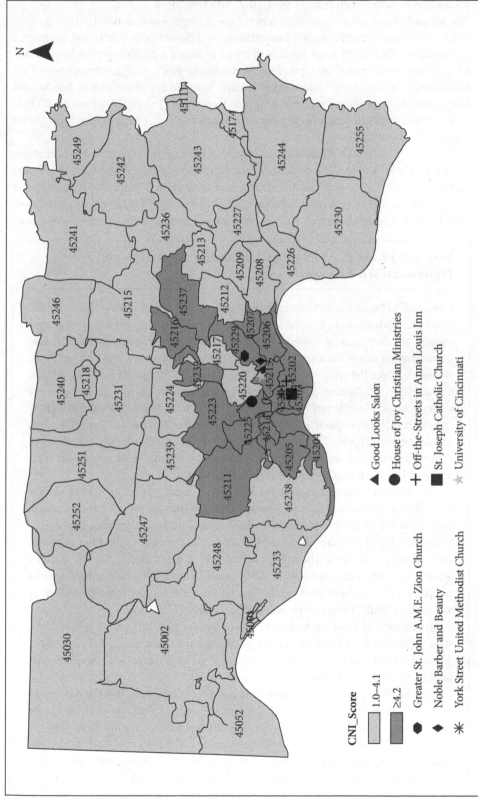

CNI_Score

◻ 1.0–4.1
▨ ≥4.2

⬟ Greater St. John A.M.E. Zion Church
◆ Noble Barber and Beauty
✳ York Street United Methodist Church

▲ Good Looks Salon
● House of Joy Christian Ministries
✛ Off-the-Streets in Anna Louis Inn
■ St. Joseph Catholic Church
★ University of Cincinnati

Figure 3.5 Community sites participating in community-engaged research.

Phase 2: Assessing Community Strengths and Dynamics

The second phase entails assessing community strengths and dynamics (Israel et al., 2013). Since community means different things to different people, it is best to obtain a definition of community from insiders. It is best to locate a community leader or stakeholder who is influential or represents a community voice and the strengths and resources of the community, including key cultural, historical, and contextual dimensions. It is preferable to conduct the interview face to face. Israel et al. (2013, Appendix D) provides a guide to developing a list of interview questions for stakeholders, including what they thinks about research.

Box 3.3 is a summary of one such interview with a Cincinnati community hairstylist stakeholder who was familiar with the community's sociopolitical and economic issues and worked for a salon that had high community influence. We selected a hairstylist at Good Looks Salon in Corryville (ZIP code: 45219), a high-need Cincinnati neighborhood. Good Looks Salon has both male barbers and female stylists and serves a diverse clientele.

Box 3.3 Phase 2: Assessing Community Strengths and Dynamics: An Example

Corryville is home to the University of Cincinnati (UC) and has diverse residents, from UC students and employees to middle-income/working-class small business owners and low-income residents. There are many government, health, and academic institutions in the area. Nearby sub-community areas are West Walnut Hills, Avondale, Over-the-Rhine (OTR), East End, West End, Prospect Hills, Mt. Auburn, and Ludlow. Mt. Auburn, home to Christ Hospital, has residential homes, grocery stores, and social service agencies. OTR has more entertainment venues and higher-income residents; people attend weekly activities on the "square." In Corryville, there are also activities for low-income persons at the community center (gym, library, rec center). Many people in some of these areas are "transitional" and some of the areas are "rough," with much poverty and limited resources.

The woman we interviewed describes each neighborhood as having similar yet varying characteristics and profiles. Parks in the area are common places where people go to convene socially. There are churches of varying denominations (Muslim, Jehovah's Witnesses, Christian). Many of the Christian churches offer activities for kids. There are many different ethnicities (Muslim, African American, German, Latino, etc.). There are different educational levels. Most people who live in these areas use the "metro" (bus) system, will ride their bikes, or will walk. Middle- to higher-income residents might have a car.

She reports that the strengths and resources of Corryville are its sports activities. With the FC Cincinnati (a U.S. professional soccer team), UC, Northern Kentucky University, and Xavier University, it is common to have "weekly" basketball, football, soccer, and track-and-field events.

Another strength of the community that she mentioned are that the businesses are supportive of one another and patronize one another. "Businesses look out for each other . . . we try to attend to making it nice, like picking up trash, planting flowers, and even starting a greenhouse garden." She also reported local community resources that she was proud of: social services; educational, economic, and volunteer opportunities; the Veterans Administration (VA); Kroger; the

Environmental Protection Agency (EPA); recreation centers; and grocery stores. Monthly community town hall meetings are well attended by business stakeholders, but not many local residents attend. She mentioned that Crossroads Health Center is largely used by low-income residents. She also spoke favorably about UC.

Safety was the first problem she described. She described this issue within the context of racial discrimination and profiling. She mentioned a 2015 incident when an unarmed African American man was fatally shot by a white UC police officer during a traffic stop for a missing front license plate and a suspended driver's license; this brought about much tension between community members and the police. "Cincinnati police are selective about who they serve and what they think is important to attend to." She feels that another weakness is the increasing costs in the area. While walking, she pointed out the increasing number of vacant and abandoned buildings and businesses in the area. She described how the price of buildings has increased, making it difficult for people to purchase vacant property.

This interview revealed that some of our preconceptions of the Corryville community were somewhat incomplete and faulty. During the interview, she was extremely open and honest about her impressions of the community and its challenges, and needs. She was insightful and was favorable about prevention and education research, particularly as it related to health, as her "mother died of cancer in her 30s." During our interview, she suggested that we take a walk in the neighborhood so that she could point out, reflect upon, and communicate issues of interest and concern. Overall, she seemed to appreciate being the local community "expert" and feeling that her voice was heard.

Phase 3: Identifying Priority Health Concerns and Research Aims

The third stage of CBPR is identifying health concerns and research aims (Israel et al., 2013). Key questions for community members and stakeholders to answer include the health concerns and problems that most impact the community. It is also important to begin to identify the causes and consequences and prioritize these community concerns. At this stage, there is often an ability to develop research aims and objectives.

We continue the example described earlier, where we engaged churches, salons, and a social service agency. During one of our community health luncheons at a partnering church, we developed a needs assessment survey where partners reported two primary health concerns: obesity and cancer. Although church leaders believe it is ideal for female congregation members to go to their physicians and providers for health information, they reported that women's health information is often obtained from their family, friends, and the media. Church leaders think the majority of women go to church leaders to discuss their health concerns (64% of those who completed the needs assessment). The data identified the top reasons that luncheon participants believed that women in their congregation and business neglect their health: cost concerns, insurance, other priorities/inconvenience/"busy," fear of a negative outcome, practical issues (work, transportation, caregiving), misconceptions ("family do not talk," "I think they will get sick in the hospital").

Stylists said they desired educational information to post on their salon websites. Stakeholders suggested the following strategies to improve women's health: "educate from the pulpit" and educational ministries, assist with insurance coverage and financial issues, and provide screenings and education while at church.

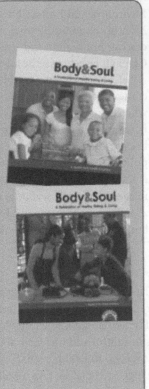

Body and Soul (National Caner Institute, 2004) is an evidence-based program that incorporates healthy lifestyle education, church events, and peer counseling and has been proven to promote healthy food choices through increased fruit and vegetable consumption.

The **primary goals** of this proposed project are: 1) to promote healthy eating among African American churches in Cincinnati zip codes with a high community need, 2) to engage these church members in the implementation of the *Body and Soul*, and 3) to implement the *Body and Soul* program in these high need Cincinnati church communities. Using community-based participatory research, we will accomplish these research goals by enrolling church leaders and members.

This proposed community-academic collaborative project – *Body and Soul*, is expected to yield insights into a culturally relevant program to encourage healthy eating behavior which can be sustainable beyond the grant period. By increasing fruits and vegetables, progress may be made toward eliminating caner and health disparities.

Figure 3.6 *Body and Soul* Program

In response to these preliminary data, we identified an intervention to adapt and test. *Body and Soul* (Resnicow et al., 2004) is an evidence-based program that incorporates healthy lifestyle education, church events, and peer counseling and has been proven to promote healthy food choices through increased fruit and vegetable consumption (Figure 3.6). Given the importance in the community and the extent of their reach, churches are effective avenues for health promotion efforts targeting African Americans (Brand, 2019; Lynch et al., 2019; Resnicow et al., 2004). This is especially important given that African Americans have higher documented mortality rates due to many diet-related diseases, like cancer (Carson et al., 2012; DeSantis et al., 2019). We can see these startling rates of disease in Cincinnati urban communities (Hoppe et al., 2019; Sastry et al., 2017). For example, when we compare data on cancer incidence and mortality nationally, in Ohio, and specifically in Cincinnati, we see an even greater burden on this region (Hoppe et al., 2019; Sastry et al., 2017). Thus, African American churches can be important centers for targeted health promotion efforts to improve dietary behavior.

Phase 4: Designing and Conducting Intervention and/or Policy Research
Based on earlier stages of identifying where to focus efforts, assessing community strengths, and identifying health needs, the next phase of CBPR involves collaboratively designing and conducting etiologic intervention and/or policy research (Israel et al., 2013). This phase entails, for example, deciding on the most appropriate research design, data

---

Box 3.4 Phase 4: Designing and Conducting Intervention Research: An Example

---

Our expert community–academic partnering team proposes an adapted version of traditional patient navigation that incorporates motivation and behavioral skills and that is specific for cervical cancer prevention, a promising strategy to reduce cervical cancer disparities among low-income African American women. Preliminary work by this team has led to the development of a novel intervention model with high potential for reducing cervical cancer disparities by increasing adherence to human papillomavirus (HPV) vaccination and cervical cancer screening and follow-up: the Navigation-Information-Motivation-Behavioral Skills (NIMBS) approach. The NIMBS expands upon the existing Information-Motivation-Behavioral (IMB) skills conceptual adherence model by combining patient navigation and IMB principles.

Though this preliminary model shows promise, further formative work is needed to understand specific barriers to cervical cancer prevention behaviors among low-income African American women in order to adapt NIMBS to address their needs. We will use the cultural adaptation process model to adapt NIMBS; cultural adaptation is a widely used method for enhancing the effectiveness of interventions by grounding them in the lived experience of the participants (Domenach-Rodriguez et al., 2010, 2012).

The primary objectives of this proposed research study are (1) to conduct formative research to theoretically and collectively understand adherence to HPV "catch-up" vaccination, regular Pap screening, and timely follow-up after abnormal Pap screens in low-income, African American women and (2) to adapt and refine the NIMBS using these data and evaluate the acceptability of the modified NIMBS. We will accomplish these objectives by enrolling low-income African American women who have not adhered to HPV vaccination and/or Pap screening or diagnostic guidelines, community stakeholders (social service agency case managers, community church leaders, hairstylists), and healthcare providers from a gynecological clinic

---

collection methods, intervention strategy, and implementation strategies (Israel et al., 2013). Box 3.4 is an example of this phase, based on preliminary work showing that the individual relevancy of information, behavioral skills (both procedural and systematic), and motivation seemed to affect women's cancer screening adherence (Wells et al., 2017).

Phase 5: Feeding Back and Interpreting Research Findings

The fifth phase is feeding back and interpreting the findings within the partnership (Israel et al., 2013). This involves sharing the findings from the research, such as the results of the analysis of the survey or the formative data results, and engaging all partners in making sense of what was found (Israel et al., 2013). This can involve an iterative process of collecting pilot data and conducting research, interpreting, and then reporting to the community. This dialog can help finetune a proposed intervention. This might mean reconvening with a community stakeholder group at another health luncheon to report on findings and obtain feedback or conducting a town hall meeting to interpret research findings.

Phase 6: Disseminating and Translating Research Findings

The sixth phase involves disseminating and translating research findings (Israel et al., 2013). Dissemination is central to academic scholarship and community translation. It is important to convert knowledge into language that a non-academic, lay audience can understand. Critical questions at this phase include:

What is the most important result to share with the community?

What are the most appropriate ways to disseminate the results to the community?

What is the role of community partners in publishing the results?

How can the results be translated and disseminated into more broad-scale interventions and policy change? (Israel et al., 2013).

Answering these questions helps solidify the working relationship into meaningful research for the community.

Phase 7: Maintaining, Sustaining, and Evaluating CBPR Partnerships

The last CBPR stage is maintaining, sustaining, and evaluating the partnership (Figure 3.7). CBPR is an ongoing process that is at the center of all these phases and occurs throughout

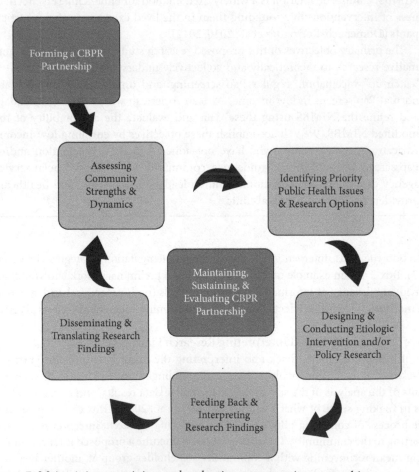

Figure 3.7 Maintaining, sustaining, and evaluating a community partnership.

each of them. Maintaining and sustaining a community partnership occurs throughout the different phases of the process; the partners work on an ongoing basis to strengthen trust, share knowledge and skills, and identify solutions as they work together to carry out the tasks involved in conducting the research. Evaluation of the community partnership also needs to start at the beginning and continue throughout the project. Relevant questions to address at this stage include:

How well is the partnership working?

How can the partnership process be improved?

What aspects of the partnership need to be considered regarding sustainability? (Israel et al., 2013).

In Box 3.5 we describe a longstanding CBPR model in St. Louis, Missouri: the Program for the Elimination of Cancer Disparities (PECaD) at the Alvin J. Siteman

---

Box 3.5 Program for the Elimination of Cancer Disparities (PECaD): An Example of All CBPR Phases

PECaD uses CBPR principles to guide its community partnerships, to inform its approach to health disparities research and outreach, and to create a framework for moving forward. The CBPR framework involves continuous communication with the community through all activities, interventions, and research, as well as reporting the results of studies they participated in back to community members. The CBPR framework also involves addressing disparities at each step, from education, screening, and diagnosis, to treatment. Through outreach and education activities, PECaD works with community partners to disseminate cancer prevention, screening, and health and wellness information to community members and organizational stakeholders. This includes sharing local research advances with community members that may benefit them; supporting and encouraging the development of local cancer interventions through our cancer site-specific community partnerships; educating underserved community gatekeepers; and developing enhancements to improve the care of underserved patients.

As implemented within the PECaD structure, CBPR entails a partnership between members of a community and academic investigators/trained experts, particularly those who experience a disproportionate burden across the cancer continuum from cancer awareness to prevention, detection, access to treatment, follow-up after therapy is completed, and survivorship. The primary focal groups included racial/ethnic minorities, residents with low socioeconomic status, and those living in rural areas or areas with limited access to healthcare. Researchers and partners have identified gaps in coverage, research priorities, and preferences. The goal is to achieve agreement on common research/programmatic problems and goals. Programs and activities use culturally competent methods developed with community representatives to increase potential reach.

Community and faculty co-chairs share leadership responsibilities. The co-chairs co-lead monthly meetings of the PECaD internal leadership team, which comprises the co-chairs, study principal investigators (PIs), training and community outreach PIs, and the project manager. The internal leadership team is responsible for guiding the implementation of PECaD programs and for translating ongoing discussion of the Disparities Elimination Advisory Committee (DEAC) into relevant programmatic plans. The DEAC oversees identification of community cancer disparity concerns that are within the PECaD capacity to respond and supports disease-specific community coalitions that obtain community and organizational input on cancer disparities that is used to initiate, implement, and evaluate activities related to issues of concern.

The Breast Cancer Community Partnership (BCaP) is the oldest of the disease-specific partnerships. BCaP remains active and is made up of cancer survivors and advocates; representatives and providers from community healthcare organizations and community-based organizations; and academic researchers, clinicians, and staff. The partnership facilitates dialog and strategic planning to address breast cancer disparities in the region. The Colorectal Cancer Community Partnership comprises community physicians, colorectal cancer (CRC) survivors, family advocates, researchers, and representatives of community-based organizations. The partnership has been in place since 2006 and works to demystify public perceptions, bridge communication gaps, and identify factors associated with navigating the system in order to obtain CRC screening.

The PECaD community health educators work to expand community outreach capacity such that cancer information is disseminated to diverse communities and is in line with the local and regional goal to eliminate cancer health disparities through community partnerships. PECaD has cancer resources in informational kiosks at regional libraries located in areas with high mortality rates and implements billboard and newspaper campaigns to increase cancer screening and prevention awareness. In addition, a Navigator Work Group received initial support from PECaD that allowed it to grow and evolve. Navigators from across the region meet to discuss challenges and ways to work around those challenges on a quarterly basis. Beyond these activities, PECaD researchers further developed and implemented a community education model for enhancing partnerships and collaborations between community and academic partners wishing to engage in CBPR. This training model provides community benefit while enhancing community members' potential to engage as equals with academic researchers. In 2013, the Community Research Fellows Training was adapted from Community Alliances for Research Empowering Social Change (CARES) program and implemented as a pilot project of the Program for the Elimination of Cancer Disparities (PECaD) at Washington University in St. Louis School of Medicine and Siteman Cancer Center (Goodman et al., 2010). The program has now graduated five cohorts, funded community pilot projects, and is expanding its reach into rural communities (Goodman & Sanders Thompson, 2017; Sanders Thompson et al., 2015).

Cancer Center of Washington University School of Medicine and Barnes-Jewish Hospital (Sanders Thompson et al., 2015; Sanders Thompson & Hood, 2016). PECaD was established in 2003 in an effort to address the excess cancer burden within the region and the state, particularly among minority and medically underserved populations. PECaD sought to create a national model for eliminating disparities in cancer through community partnerships and CBPR. Primary efforts focused on the most common cancers, including breast, lung, prostate, and colorectal cancer, among African Americans and low-income people. This exemplar best illustrates the circular (rather than linear) CBPR process addressing cancer disparities.

Summary

Ultimately, CBPR is an approach to research that is about advancing change to improve health and well-being in communities through community partnerships. It represents a paradigm shift from traditional models of addressing cancer disparities and inequities. As we look ahead in the future of cancer prevention and control, we must look toward CBPR solutions that go beyond healthcare providers in the clinic or hospital. And in research, we need to go beyond community-placed research in order to better apply CBPR definitions, frameworks, and evidence-based strategies. Healthcare professionals and academic institutions need to partner with community stakeholders to address some of these inequities. With a genuine interest in pursuing public health change, communities in need will be more willing to "give voice" in working with academics and healthcare providers to develop, implement, and disseminate meaningful solutions.

References

Agency for Healthcare Research and Quality. (2017). Effective health care program stakeholder guide. http://www.ahrq.gov/clinic/epcpartner/stakeholderguide/

Boeshart, T., & Carlson, E. D. (2014). Hamilton County maternal and infant health monthly surveillance report. *Available from:) Hamilton County Public Health, Department of Community Health Services, Division of Epidemiology and Assessment in collaboration with Cradle Cincinnati.*

Brand, D. J. (2019). Barriers and facilitators of faith-based health programming within the African American church. *Journal of Cultural Diversity, 26*(1), 3–8.

Burke, J. G., Hess, S., Hoffmann, K., Guizzetti, L., Loy, E., Gielen, A., Bailey, M., Walnoha, A., Barbee, G., & Yonas, M. (2013). Translating community-based participatory research principles into practice. *Progress in Community Health Partnerships: Research, Education, and Action, 7*(2), 115–122. doi:10.1353/cpr.2013.0025

Carson, J. S., Michalsky, L., Latson, B., Banks, K., Tong, L., Gimpel, N., Lee, J. J., & DeHaven, M. J. (2012). The cardiovascular health of urban African Americans: Diet-related results from the Genes, Nutrition, Exercise, Wellness, and Spiritual Growth (GoodNEWS) trial. *Journal of the Academy of Nutrition and Dietetics, 112*(11), 1852–1858.

Centers for Disease Control and Prevention, Public Health Practice Program Office. (1997). Principles of community engagement.

CityLink Center. (2018). Poverty in Cincinnati. https://citylinkcenter.org/about-us/the-need/poverty-in-cincinnati

De Koning, K., & Martin, M. (Eds.) (1996). *Participatory research in health: Issues and experiences.* Zed Books.

DeSantis, C. E., Miller, K. D., Sauer, A. G., Jemal, A., & Siegel, R. L. (2019). Cancer statistics for African Americans, 2019. *CA: A Cancer Journal for Clinicians, 69*(3), 211.

Domenech-Rodriguez, M., Baumann, A., & Schwartz, A. (2010). Cultural adaptation of an evidence based intervention: From theory to practice in a Latino/a community context. *American Journal of Community Psychology, 47*, 170–186.

Domenech-Rodriguez, M., & Bernal, G. (2012). Frameworks, models, and guidelines for cultural adaptation. In G. Bernal & M. Domenech-Rodriguez (Eds.), *Cultural adaptations*. American Psychological Association, 23–40.

Fals-Borda, O., & Rahman, M. (Eds.). (1991). *Action and knowledge: Breaking the monopoly with participatory action research*. Apex.

Goodman, M. S., Dias, J. J., & Stafford, J. D. (2010). Increasing research literacy in minority communities: CARES fellows training program. *Journal of Empirical Research on Human Research Ethics, 5*(4), 33–41.

Goodman, M. S., & Sanders Thompson, V. (2017). *Public health research methods for partnerships and practice*. CRC Press, Taylor & Francis Group.

Health Collaborative. (2016). Community health needs assessment: A regional collaborative report. https://cmhcinc.org/wp-content/uploads/2018/12/Cincinnati-CHNA-Report-2016-FINAL-1-5-16MD.pdf

Hills, M., Mullett, J., & Carroll, S. (2007). Community-based participatory action research: Transforming multidisciplinary practice in primary health care. *Revista Panamericana Salud Publica, 21*(2/3), 125–135.

Hoppe, E. J., Hussain, L. R., Grannan, K. J., Dunki-Jacobs, E. M., Lee, D. Y., & Wexelman, B. A. (2019). Racial disparities in breast cancer persist despite early detection: Analysis of treatment of stage 1 breast cancer and effect of insurance status on disparities. *Breast Cancer Research and Treatment, 173*(3), 597–602.

International Collaboration for Participatory Health Research (ICPHR). (2013). *Position paper 1: What is participatory health research?* International Collaboration for Participatory Health Research.http://www.icphr.org/position-papers—discussion-papers/position-paper-no-1

Irwin, A. (1995). *Citizen science: A study of people, expertise and sustainable development*. Routledge.

Israel, B. A. (2013). *Methods for community-based participatory research for health*. Jossey-Bass.

Israel, B. A., Coombe, C. M., Cheezum, R. R., Schulz, A. J., McGranaghan, R. J., Lichtenstein, R., Reyes, A. G., Clement, J., & Burris, A. (2010). Community-based participatory research: A capacity-building approach for policy advocacy aimed at eliminating health disparities. *American Journal of Public Health, 100*(11), 2094–2102. doi:10.2105/AJPH.2009.170506

Israel, B. A., Schulz, A. J., Parker, E. A., & Becker, A. B. (2001). Community-based participatory research: Policy recommendations for promoting a partnership approach in health research. *Education for Health, 14*(2), 182–197. http://web.a.ebscohost.com/ehost/pdfviewer/pdfviewer?vid=0&sid=7be524bf-b65d-49d1-9b7a-59afb65fe3a2%40sessionmgr4007

Israel, A. B., Schultz, A. J., Parker, E. A., & Becker, A. B (1998). Review of community-based research: Assessing partnership approaches to improve public health. *Annual Review of Public Health, 19*, 173– 202.

Jason, L. A., Keys, C. B., Suarez-Balcazar, Y., Taylor, R. R., & Davis, M. I. (Eds.). (2004). *Participatory community research: Theories and methods in action*. American Psychological Association. http://dx.doi.org/10.1037/10726-000

Jones, L. (2009). Preface: Community-partnered participatory research: how we can work together to improve community health. *Ethnicity & Disease, 19*(4 Suppl 6), 1–2.

Knudsen, K. (2017). Zip codes vs. genetic code: Breaking down cancer disparities in Philadelphia. https://www.phillyvoice.com/Zip-code-genetics-breakdown-cancer-disparities-Philadelphia/

Kumar, J., Kidd, T., Li, Y., Lindshield, E., Muturi, N., & Adhikari, K. (2014). Using the community-based participatory research (CBPR) approach in childhood obesity prevention. *International Journal of Child Health and Nutrition, 3*, 170–178.

Lynch, E., Emery-Tiburco, E., Dugan, S., Stark White, F., Thomason, C., Jenkins, L., Feit, C., Avery-Mamer, E., Wang, Y., Mack, L., & Ragland, A. (2019). Results of ALIVE: A faith-based pilot intervention to improve diet among African American church members. *Progress in Community Health Partnerships: Research, Education, and Action, 3*(1), 19–30.

McLeroy, K. R., Bibeau, D., Steckler, A., & Glanz, K. (1988). An ecological perspective on health promotion programs. *Health Education & Behavior, 15*(4), 351–377.

Pyrch, T. (1991). Action and knowledge: Breaking the monopoly with participatory action research. Orlando Fals-Borda and Mohammad Anisur Rahman (Eds.) 1991. Apex Press.

Canadian Journal for the Study of Adult Education, 5(2), 66–71.

Reason, P., & Rowan, J. (1981). *Human inquiry: A sourcebook of new paradigm research.* Wiley.

Resnicow, K., Campbell, M. K., Carr, C., McCarty, F., Wang, T., Periasamy, S., Rahotep, S., Doyle, C., Williams, A., & Stables, G. (2004). Body and soul: A dietary intervention conducted through African American churches. *American Journal of Preventive Medicine 27*(2), 97–105.

Rifkin, S. B. (1996). Paradigms lost: Toward a new understanding of community participation in health programmes. *Acta Tropica, 61*(2), 79–92.

Sanders Thompson, V. L., Drake, B., James, A. S., Norfolk, M., Goodman, M., Ashford, L., Jackson, S., Witherspoon, M., Brewster, M., & Colditz, G. (2015). A community coalition to address cancer disparities: Transitions, successes and challenges. *Journal of Cancer Education, 30*(4), 616–622.

Sanders Thompson, V. L., & Hood, S. L. (2016). Academic and community partnerships and social change. In W. F. Tate IV, N. Staudt, & A. Macrander (Eds.), *The crisis of race in higher education: A day of discovery and dialogue.* Emerald Group Publishing Limited, 127–149.

Sastry, S., Zoller, H. M., Walker, T., & Sunderland, S. (2017). From patient navigation to cancer justice: Toward a culture-centered, community-owned intervention addressing disparities in cancer prevention. *Frontiers in Communication, 2*, 1–12.

Smithies, J., & Webster, G. (1998). *Community involvement in health: From passive recipients to active participants.* Ashgate.

Stokols, D. (1996). Translating social ecological theory into guidelines for community health promotion. *American Journal of Health Promotion, 10*(4), 282–298.

Tapp, H., White, L., Steuerwald, M., & Dulin, M. (2013). Use of community-based participatory research in primary care to improve healthcare outcomes and disparities in care. *Journal of Comparative Effectiveness Research, 2*(4), 405–419. doi:10.2217/cer.13.45

Wells, A., Shon, E., McGowan, K., & James, A. (2017). Perspectives of low-income African American women non-adherent to mammography screening: The importance of information, behavioral skills, and motivation. *Journal of Cancer Education, 32*(2), 328–334.

Wells, A., Thompson, V., Yeakey, C., Ross, W., & Notaro, S. (2019). *Poverty and Place: Cancer Prevention among Low Income Women of Color.* Plymouth, UK: Lexington Books, Inc.: Public Health Series.

Whyte, W. F. (Ed.). (1991). *Participatory action research.* Sage Publications, Inc.

Chapter 3 Takeaways

- Self-awareness of culture, biases, and worldviews on the part of healthcare providers is the critical first step toward conceptualizing an evaluation that will garner buy-in from the community, capitalize on strengths, and mitigate vulnerabilities. Engagement with stakeholders throughout the evaluation process is vital.

- Community-based participatory research (CBPR) is an approach to research that is about advancing change to improve health and well-being in communities through community partnerships. As we look ahead in the future of cancer prevention and control, we must look toward CBPR solutions (not merely community-placed research) that go beyond healthcare providers in the clinic or hospital. Healthcare professionals and academic institutions need to partner with community stakeholders; such partnerships will likely result in more willingness of communities to "give voice" in developing, implementing, and disseminating meaningful solutions to addressing cancer disparities and inequities among low-income women of color.

Conclusion

Cancer Navigation: Charting the Path Forward for Low-Income Women of Color is an attempt to address health inequities at a provider and healthcare system level. We have discussed the social and structural barriers (e.g., high unemployment and poverty rates, lack of insurance, poor transportation infrastructure, and lower levels of patient education) that preclude low-income women of color from reaching their full health potential. Thus, multilevel strategies that can translate into improved access are necessary to improve population health. Students and professional and lay providers play an important role in addressing the social determinants of health that contribute to such health inequities. Thus, our mission in this book was to educate students and providers about the multiple levels of healthcare inequities, their impact, and practical skills and actions that might address them. This concluding chapter provides a summary of the book.

We discussed a partnership in care that begins with a basic understanding of the barriers and stressors faced by low-income women, culturally competent communication and engagement, and evidence-based interventions and strategies important to treatment across the cancer continuum. We ended this work with an examination of the relevance of evaluation of interventions and programs designed or adapted to meet the unique needs of diverse low-income women.

Delivering patient-centered care is fundamentally the goal of the chronic care model (CCM) and other models that promote chronic disease self-management. Inherent in the philosophy of patient-centered care is the high priority placed on an individual's specific health needs and desired health outcomes. Consequently, medical decision-making in a patient-centered care approach embraces a patient's beliefs and values toward well-being, which becomes the driving force behind all healthcare decisions and quality measurements. A hallmark of high-quality care for low-income women with cancer is the delivery of patient-centered care in a manner that is collaborative, coordinated, and accessible. This book has provided robust examples of how cancer care in low-income settings can still be collaborative and highly coordinated. However, accessibility of care, a cardinal feature of the CCM, is not universally assured for low-income women.

Summary of the Introduction

In Module I.1, "Cancer 101," we began to understand the "knowns and unknowns" of cancer. Because many health inequities actually grow out of a lack of understanding, we began with a focus on four of the most common cancers that affect low-income women of color: lung cancer, breast cancer, colorectal cancer, and cervical cancer. We discussed preventive health behaviors, health behaviors that reduce cancer risk, and screening and early detection methods for each of these cancers. We provided a flowchart for each of these cancers based on American Cancer Society (2016, 2017, 2018, 2019) screening

Cancer Navigation. Anjanette A. Wells, Vetta L. Sanders Thompson, Will Ross, Carol Camp Yeakey, and Sheri R. Notaro,
Oxford University Press. © Oxford University Press 2022. DOI: 10.1093/med/9780190672867.003.0005

guidelines. These graphical representations easily explain the screening criteria and process for patients who may not understand screening. To our knowledge, however, these flowcharts are absent from the literature.

In Module I.2, "Chronic Care Conceptual Model," we contextualized the entire approach to this book by introducing the expanded CCM (Barr et al., 2003), which includes components critical for increasing access, health delivery redesign, and development and implementation of policies designed to improve population health. Multiple studies have confirmed that uninsured and underinsured cancer patients have worse outcomes than patients who are insured (Ayanian et al., 1993; Brookfield, 2009; Fedewa & Ahn, 2011; Ou, 2008). The Affordable Care Act (ACA) was the most recent attempt to redesign the delivery model in order to improve healthcare access. Under ACA, the number of uninsured nonelderly Americans decreased from over 44 million in 2013 (the year before the major coverage provisions went into effect) to just below 27 million in 2016. In 2017, the number of uninsured people increased by nearly 700,000 people, the first increase since implementation of the ACA. Most uninsured people are in low-income families in which there is at least one worker. Individuals below the poverty line are at the highest risk of being uninsured (Dickman et al., 2017) In total, more than eight in 10 of uninsured people were in families with incomes below 400% of the poverty line in 2017. But the number of *underinsured* Americans has steadily climbed, increasing from approximately 29 million in 2010 to 44 million in 2018 (Collins et al., 2019).

Summary of Chapter 1

In Module 1.1, "Cancer Communication," we noted that communication is a key issue in efforts to meet the cancer care needs of low-income women of color. Health literacy is a major factor in the process, but there are many other issues as women begin to make decisions about screening and preventive behaviors and move on to care and survivorship if there is a cancer diagnosis. Providers must pay close attention to the language they use. Jargon-free, plain language is a start, but they must also consider the patient's first and preferred language, dialects, and culturally relevant terminology and colloquialisms. All providers and staff should know when translators and interpreters are available and how to contact them. Providers must be willing to engage in patient-centered care that makes time for explanations, questions, and support. Simplicity is key in both verbal and written communications. Directions for care, summaries of treatments and medications, and clear action steps to support health should be readily available to patients, and an effort should be made to assess their understanding. Those who produce health information materials must also consider these issues and should include visual elements and designs that meet patients' literacy needs as well as those that suggest inclusion and cultural competence. The provider community, from physicians to community navigators, must select information with community norms, needs, and access in mind. If culturally appropriate materials are not available, cultural adaptation of existing materials must consider and adhere to standards outlined in the literature and described in Chapter 1.

Module 1.2, "Recognizing and Assessing Adherence Barriers and Stressors," provided profiles of low-income women of color and discussed the full range of factors that can get in the way of preventive screening and cancer care for this population. The challenges that many of these women face can make it difficult to follow up with care and include financial strain, insurance concerns, housing problems, physical and mental health issues, legal problems, caregiving demands, underemployment or unemployment, employment commitments, and problems accessing healthcare systems. We also described another category of barriers that are not often discussed: organizational barriers, such as mistreatment by providers and discrimination. These real-world barriers and stressors were brought to life in two highlighted cases. "If . . . then" statements were listed to suggest possible responses for the provider when assisting a patient to overcome barriers.

Module 1.3, "Culturally Competent Communication, Assessment, and Engagement," discussed the relevance and importance of cultural competency in communication, assessment, and engagement with patients. Particularly with practice among low-income women of color, their lived experiences are descriptors of intersectionality. This is why we must first have an awareness, acceptance, and knowledge of difference. This module discussed diverse racial/ethnic, religious, and socioeconomic populations. Of course, the discussion did not capture all populations of low-income women of color, as there is diversity based on gender, age, sexual orientation, disability, immigration status, and other important characteristics and identifications.

Summary of Chapter 2

Module 2.1, "Patient Navigation," started with a discussion of the importance of patient navigation for women of color and covered the ingredients and skills needed to implement a patient navigation program. As shown in Wells et al. (2019), we have found that when attempting to encourage nonadherent or hard-to-reach women to initiate and maintain cancer screening, it is most important to focus on four areas: problem solving, information, motivation, and behaviors.

Module 2.2, "Survivorship Care Plans," highlighted the increased use of these plans, which is an important development in cancer care. However, merely producing these plans is insufficient; to be of value to low-income women of color, the plans must be shared with the patient and the primary care provider. Patients and families should have an opportunity to discuss and problem solve any troubling aspects of the plan before making the transition away from oncology care. Navigators should take into account socioeconomic and cultural barriers to care, as well as resources for medical care and financial and emotional support that are available in the community. Strategies and resources to achieve "warm hand-offs," as the patient's care transitions to healthcare providers in the community, should be explored and included in the survivorship care plan. The module concluded with a sample survivorship care plan modified to include cultural and socioecological areas of relevance for low-income women of color.

Module 2.3, "Clinical Trial Uptake: Additional Options for Treatment," discussed clinical trials, an option that sometimes broadens cancer treatment options. Clinical trials may represent a significant opportunity to improve cancer health equity among low-income women of color. We discussed the problem of clinical trial underrepresentation among women and persons of color and the barriers to inclusion and participation. We concluded by illustrating four common scenarios that we might see in real-world practice, with possible interpersonal strategies to encourage participation.

Summary of Chapter 3

Module 3.1, "Outcomes and Assessing Intervention Efforts," explored the complex topic of evaluating interventions within a health equity framework. Several examples from the evidence-based public health (EBPH) literature were provided to illustrate the importance of considering whether the outcomes of programs and interventions differ for underrepresented or marginalized communities. One intervention that illustrated the challenges in framing evaluation within a health equity lens focused on a program designed to improved self-regulation skills for low-income individuals receiving employment services through the federal program Temporary Assistance for Needy Families (TANF) (e.g., Hardy, 2019; Kautz et al., 2014). Self-regulation skills include the ability to stay organized, control emotions, complete tasks, and persevere.

Module 3.2, "Community-Based Participatory Research," included some examples from our work in Cincinnati, Ohio, highlighting the role that community engagement can play in promoting cancer health and preventive behaviors. The premise is that community members are more likely to accept cancer screening, health preventive behaviors, and treatment recommendations when they have the opportunity to provide input. Such input may relate to the use of available resources, design style and language, and channel and media selection to broaden exposure and uptake. In addition, the information provided as a part of community education may influence community norms in ways that increase support for cancer screening and health behaviors. This information may strategically focus on misinformation, fears, and emotional concerns as well as legitimate community mistrust based on healthcare system and provider relationships with segments or specific populations in the community. The most important issue in community engagement is to show respect for the community and respect for the wisdom and knowledge that lives there. There are many strategies for engaging communities. It is important for healthcare systems and providers to be innovative to meet the needs of the community. Whatever strategy is selected to increase cancer preventive behavior, treatment, and survivorship, there must be inclusion of diverse voices, consideration of community context, and clear benefit to the patients and community served.

Future Research

With the explosion of research (and funding) of precision medicine, we must also use a broader lens to improve the health of low-income women. Due to the disparities in cancer diagnosis, treatment, and mortality rates, patients who are most affected by cancer are often the ones with the least access to precision medicine studies (Fiscella, 2004; Marcus, 2016). Examples of precision medicine approaches include examining targeted therapies for triple-negative breast cancer in Black women and advancing research on biological explanations for why Black men are more likely to die of prostate cancer than White men (Vadaparampil et al., 2017). Full implementation of the expanded CCM will undoubtedly improve the overall health of low-income women living with cancer. But it is important to understand that this model cannot be successful with low-income women of color unless we receive support at a policy level.

Conclusion

As we conclude this volume, we begin to understand that there are several ways to re-configure the healthcare system to more effectively deliver care to low-income women. Strategies of interest include increasing the number of community health workers and cancer navigators and reforming the payment system to emphasize performance. Ultimately, true and effective healthcare delivery and redesign must focus on reducing the number of uninsured and underinsured. In a sign of progress, in the 2018 midterm elections voters in Idaho, Nebraska, and Utah passed Medicaid expansions, joining 33 states that had previously done so. At the time of this writing, Missouri, which had been one of 13 states that had not expanded Medicaid, did so through an initiative on the August 2020 ballot.

We believe that an integrated approach is needed to move toward cancer and health equity, and the expanded CCM provides such an approach. This model is not just a theory but represents a practical strategy that providers can use in real-world practice. It is important for us to realize that solutions to addressing cancer and other health inequities must also come from multiple levels: individuals, providers, wraparound services, and local grassroots organizations who take it upon themselves to work for a greater good. We need safe community venues and places that can bring people together as a means to educate others, where we can build community wisdom, resources, and capacity into something that will ensure that we all have the opportunity for good health.

The COVID-19 pandemic has unveiled fissures in American society that represent the country's failure to confront racism in all its forms. Some 52 years ago, the bipartisan U.S. National Advisory Commission on Civil Disorders (known as the Kerner Commission) researched and analyzed the causes of over 150 race-related riots in 1967. One of the main conclusions of its 1968 report was that America was "moving toward two societies, one black and one white—separate and unequal."

Consider:

- More than 300,000 people have died from COVID-19, a disease that has disproportionately killed people of color because of systemic racism.
- Police were called on Christian Cooper, an African American male who was birdwatching in Central Park.
- A woman attacked a 14-year-old youth in a New York City hotel, in the presence of his parent, as he was accused of stealing his own cellphone.
- George Floyd, Ahmaud Arbery, Breonna Taylor, Eric Garner, Michael Brown, Philando Castile, Tamir Rice, Walter Scott, Atatiana Jefferson, Alton Sterling, Trayvon Martin, and so many others over the years who have been killed by the police and others.

These events are compounded by the racism that is baked into our institutions for the benefit of those who hold power and privilege. As Mitch Landrieu wrote in the *New York Times* in June 2020:

What is called for is a redesign of the systems that have keep America divided for generations: from the housing system that continues to segregate; a criminal justice system designed to keep persons of color "under control"; an economy that benefits the top

1% at the benefit of workers we only now deem "essential"; an education system that educates the rich at the expense of the poor; a political system designed to make voting a privilege and not a right; and a health care system that leaves too many without care.

The coronavirus has been anything but a great equalizer. It has been the great revealer, pulling back the curtain on the class and racial divide in America. It is time to take this opportunity to look at the broken systems that perpetuate this growing inequality. Addressing the uneven distribution of opportunity and wealth and the provision of affordable healthcare sufficient to one's needs would be a good starting point.

Quality healthcare does not just affect patients. It also affects healthcare providers and all those who work in clinics and healthcare organizations, as well as their families. The reality is that the healthcare system affects everyone. As Dr. Martin Luther King Jr. said in 1966, in the opening quote to this volume, "injustice in health is the most shocking and inhumane" form of inequality. We concur. In compiling this volume, we have attempted to convey what has become a universal truism—that real wealth is good health. The day on which we become silent about those for whom good health is a privilege instead of a fundamental right is the day on which we fail all of humanity.

References

American Cancer Society. (2018). American Cancer Society guideline for colorectal cancer screening. https://www.cancer.org/cancer/colon-rectal-cancer/detection-diagnosis-staging/acs-recommendations.html

American Cancer Society. (2017). American Cancer Society recommendations for the early detection of breast cancer. https://www.cancer.org/cancer/breast-cancer/screening-tests-and-early-detection/american-cancer-society-recommendations-for-the-early-detection-of-breast-cancer.html

American Cancer Society. (2019). Lung cancer. https://www.cancer.org/cancer/lung-cancer.html

American Cancer Society. (2016). Tests for cervical cancer. https://www.cancer.org/cancer/cervical-cancer/detection-diagnosis-staging/how-diagnosed.html

Ayanian, J. Z., Kohler B. A., Abe T., & Epstein, A. M. (1993).The relation between health insurance coverage and clinical outcomes among women with breast cancer. *New England Journal of Medicine, 329,* 326–331. 10.1056/NEJM199307293290507

Barr, V., Robinson, S., Marin-Link, B., Underhill, L., Dotts, A., Ravensdale, D., & Salivaras, S. (2003). The expanded chronic care model: An integration of concepts and strategies from population health promotion and the chronic care model. *Hospital Quarterly, 7*(1), 73–82.

Brookfield, S. (2009). The concept of critical reflection: Promises and contradictions. *European Journal of Social Work, 12*(3), 293–304. doi:10.1080/13691450902945215

Collins, S. R., Bhupal, H. K., & Doty, M. M. (2019). Health insurance coverage eight years after the ACA: Fewer uninsured americans and shorter coverage gaps, but more underinsured. *Commonwealth Fund,* Feb. 2019. https://doi.org/10.26099/penv-q932

Dickman, S. L., Himmelstein, D. U., & Woolhandler, S. (2017). Inequality and the healthcare system in the USA. *The Lancet, 389*(10077), 1431–1441. https://doi.org/10.1016/s0140-6736(17)30398-7

Fedewa, A. L., & Ahn, S. (2011). The effects of physical activity and physical fitness on children's achievement and cognitive outcomes: A meta-analysis. *Research Quarterly for Exercise and Sport, 82,* 521–535. doi:10.1080/02701367.2011.10599785

Fiscella, K., Meldrum, S., Franks, P., Shields, C. G., Duberstein, P., McDaniel, S. H., & Epstein, R. M. (2004). Patient trust. *Medical Care, 42*(11), 1049–1055. https://doi.org/10.1097/00005650-200411000-00003

Hardy, B. L., Samudra, R., & Davis, J. A. (2019). Cash assistance in America: The role of race, politics, and poverty. *The Review of Black Political Economy, 46*(4), 306–324. https://doi.org/10.1177/0034644619865272

Kautz, T., & Moore, Q. (2018). Measuring self-regulation skills in evaluations of employment programs for low-income populations: Challenges and recommendations. OPRE Report #2018-83. https://www.acf.hhs.gov/opre/report/measuring-self-regulation-skills-evaluations-employment-programs-low-income-populations

Landrieu, M. (June 3, 2020). The price we have paid for not confronting racism. *New York Times.* https://www.nytimes.com/2020/06/03/opinion/george-floyd-protest-racism.html

Marcus, P. M., Pashayan, N., Church, T. R., Doria-Rose, V. P., Gould, M. K., Hubbard, R. A., Marrone, M., Miglioretti, D. L., Pharoah, P. D., Pinsky, P. F., Rendle, K. A., Robbins, H. A., Roberts, M. C., Rolland, B., Schiffman, M., Tiro, J. A., Zauber, A. G., Winn, D. M., & Khoury, M. J. (2016, November 1). *Population-based precision cancer screening: A symposium on evidence, epidemiology, and next steps.* Cancer Epidemiology, Biomarkers & Prevention. https://cebp.aacrjournals.org/content/25/11/1449.

U.S. National Advisory Commission on Civil Disorders. (1968). *Kerner report.* U.S. Government Printing Office.

Ou, S.-H. I., Zell, J. A., Ziogas, A., & Anton-Culver, H. (2008). Low socioeconomic status is a poor prognostic factor for survival in stage i nonsmall cell lung cancer and is independent of surgical treatment, race, and marital status. *Cancer, 112*(9), 2011–2020. https://doi.org/10.1002/cncr.23397

Vadaparampil, S. T., Christie, J., Donovan, K. A., Kim, J., Augusto, B., Kasting, M. L., Holt, C. L., Ashing, K., Halbert, C. H., & Pal, T. (2017). Health-related quality of life in Black breast cancer survivors with and without triple-negative breast cancer (TNBC). *Breast Cancer Research and treatment, 163*(2), 331–342. https://doi.org/10.1007/s10549-017-4173-0

Wells, A., Thompson, V., Yeakey, C., Ross, W., & Notaro, S. (2019). *Poverty and Place: Cancer Prevention among Low Income Women of Color.* Plymouth, UK: Lexington Books, Inc.: Public Health Series.

Index

Tables, figures, and boxes are indicated by *t*, *f*, and *b* following the page number

adherence barriers and stressors
  among low-income women of color, 47–50
  to breast cancer treatment, 45–47
  case study 1, 50–52, 50*b*, 51*f*
  case study 2, 52–54, 52*b*, 54*f*
  overcoming with information, 91–92
  overview of, 168–169
  poverty profiles of low-income women, 54–66
  recognizing, 43–45
  role of communication and
    engagement, 30–31
Affordable Care Act (ACA), 86, 168
African Americans
  changing demographics among, 76
  COVID-19 pandemic and, 3
  CRC (colorectal cancer) screening and, 33–39
  effectiveness of CCM for, 24
  higher risk of colorectal cancer among, 11
  interpersonal barriers and, 126
  mortality due to diet-related diseases, 158
  pediatric emergency department visits due to
    asthma, 146
  preterm and low birth weight in, 75–76
  underrepresentation in clinical trials, 123–124
African American women
  acknowledging racism and sexism when
    working with, 80
  adherence barriers to breast cancer
    treatment, 45–47
  breast cancer mortality among, 1
  cervical cancer incidence and death, 8–9
  cervical cancer screening and, 159
  effectiveness of CCM for, 24, 27, 139
  five-year relative cancer survival rate, 112
  intersectionality and, 74–75
  patient navigation and, 86
  poverty rates among, 76
  rates of obesity among, 115
  sense of community among, 150–151
American Cancer Society (ACS)
  "Cancer Facts and Figures," 1
  cancer screening guidelines, 10*t*, 167–168
  survivorship care plans (SCPs), 115
American Evaluation Association, 139–140
American Society for Clinical Oncology (ASCO),
  114–115
anti-immigrant bias, 73
Armenian beliefs and practices, 78
ASCO (American Society for Clinical Oncology),
  survivorship care plans (SCPs), 114–115

Baha'i beliefs and practices, 78
Baptist beliefs and practices, 78
barriers, definition of term, 8*t*. *See also* adherence
    barriers and stressors
BCaP (Breast Cancer Community Partnership), 162*b*
bias
  definition of term, 81*t*
  implicit bias, 73
bigotry, definition of term, 81*t*
biological literacy, 33
Black Muslim beliefs and practices, 78
Body and Soul program, 158, 158*f*
BPHC (Bureau of Primary Health Care), 19
breast cancer
  adherence barriers to breast cancer treatment, 45–47
  causes of and risk factors for, 9
  description of, 9
  incidence among women of color, 8
  mortality in African American women, 1
  overcoming barriers to screening, 91–92
  preventing, 10*t*
  screening recommendations, 12*t*, 13–14, 13*f*
Breast Cancer Community Partnership (BCaP), 162*b*
Buddhist churches of America, 78
Bureau of Primary Health Care (BPHC), 19

cancer
  among low-income women of color, 8–9
  causes of and risk factors for, 9–11
  definition of term, 7
  overcoming barriers to screening, 91–92
  pre- and posttests, 7, 17*t*
  preventing, 10*t*
  screening recommendations, 10*t*, 11–17, 12*f*, 12*t*,
    13*f*, 15*f*, 16*f*
  types of, 9
cancer disparities, definition of term, 8*t*. *See also*
    health disparities
cancer knowledge pretest, 7*t*
cancer-related terms, 8*t*
carcinogens, definition of term, 8*t*
care model. *See* chronic care model (CCM)
CBPR. *See* community-based participatory research
    (CBPR)
Center for Culturally Responsive Evaluation and
    Assessment (CREA), 147
Centers for Disease Control and Prevention (CDC)
  Funding Opportunity Announcements, 137
  model for program evaluation, 139–148, 140*f*
  survivorship care plans (SCPs), 115

cervical cancer
among African American women, 159
causes of and risk factors for, 11
deaths due to, 8–9
preventing, 10t
screening recommendations, 12t, 16, 16f
change talk, 93
chronic care model (CCM), 4, 19–27, 167–168
components of, 21t
concepts and components, 26–27t
conceptual framework, 23f
diagram of, 20f
goal of, 167
as implemented for mammography screenings, 24t
integrating population health using expanded CCM, 25f
overview of, 168
chronic stress, 48
Church of Jesus Christ of Latter-day Saints, 78
CLAS (culturally and linguistically appropriate services), 77
clinical trials
absence of diverse populations in, 123
barriers to participation, 125–127
communication storyboards, 127–131
opportunities afforded by, 123
overview of, 169
underrepresentation by specific subgroups, 123–125
underrepresentation of low-income women of color in, 8
CNI (Community Needs Index), 153b
colorectal cancer (CRC)
causes of and risk factors for, 9–11
communication and engagement for screening and treatment of, 33–39, 35f, 36f
description of, 9
preventing, 10t
screening recommendations, 12t, 14–15, 15f
communication and engagement. See also
adherence barriers and stressors; cultural competency
for colorectal cancer, 33–39, 35f
communication tips, 40b
engagement reminder checklist, 95f
health communication planning process, 36f
health literacy, 31–33, 34b
key points, 84
as key to adherence and health outcomes, 30–31
overview of, 168–169
stakeholder engagement in program evaluation, 140–141
communication storyboards, 127–131
community-based participatory research (CBPR), 149–163, 151f, 170
assessing community strengths and dynamics, 156–157, 156–157b
Body and Soul program, 158f
community sites participating, 155f
community stakeholders, 151
definition of CBPR, 149–150
definition of community, 150–151
designing and conducting intervention research, 159b
focusing research efforts, 153, 153b
forming partnerships through engagement, 154, 154b
identifying priority health concerns and research aims, 157–158
key principles of, 150
maintaining, sustaining, and evaluating CBPR partnerships, 160f
overview of, 170
phases of, 152–163
program for elimination of cancer disparities, 161–162b
social ecological model, 152
community engaged evaluation. See program evaluation
Community Needs Index (CNI), 153b
COVID-19 pandemic, 2–3, 34b, 171–172
Crenshaw, Kimberlé Williams, 74
cultural awareness, 80
cultural blindness, definition of, 81t
cultural competency
applying to intersectional identities and needs, 74–75
concepts of, 81–82t
concepts of difference in health, 75–77
cultural awareness, 80
cultural humility, 78–80
culturally competent practitioners, 72
cultural sensitivity, 80
definition of, 72, 81t
as essential for successful interventions, 71
importance to low-income women of color, 72–73
overview of, 169
in practice, 73–74
in program evaluation, 139–148
role of culture, 71
standards for appropriate services, 77
cultural humility, 78–80
culturally and linguistically appropriate services (CLAS), 77
cultural practices, 78–80
cultural sensitivity, 80
cultural values and beliefs, 71
culture, definition of term, 72, 81t

data analysis, components of, 146
data collection instruments, 143–144
discrimination
definition of, 81t
intersectionality and, 74–75
discrimination stress, 49–50
Disparities Elimination Advisory Committee (DEAC), 162b
diversity, definition of, 81t

effectiveness trials, 138
efficacy trials, 138
engagement reminder checklist, 95*f*
ethnicity, definition of, 81*t*
evaluation. *See* program evaluation
evidence-based public health (EBPH), 137–139, 139*f*, 170

fatalism
    as barrier to breast cancer screening, 46
    as barrier to CRC (colorectal cancer) screening, 33
    definition of, 81*t*
federally qualified health centers, definition of term, 8*t*
formative evaluations, 143
Freeman, Harold, 86
Funding Opportunity Announcements, 137
future research, 170

genetic, definition of term, 8*t*
genetic risk, 8*t*, 9

health disparities
    cultural competency and, 75–77
    definition of, 81*t*
Health Disparities Cancer Collaboratives (HDCC), 19–20
health equity
    cultural competency and, 75
    culturally and linguistically appropriate services (CLAS), 77
    evaluating interventions, 170
    focus of, 1–2
    improving through clinical trials, 123, 169
    increasing through CBPR, 149
health literacy, 31–33, 34*b*
high-risk, hard-to-reach populations, 97–99, 99*f*
Hispanic Americans
    cervical cancer incidence and death, 8
    changing demographics among, 76
    intersectionality and, 74
    poverty among Hispanic women, 76
    preterm and low birth weight in, 75–76
    underrepresentation in clinical trials, 123–124
homophobia, definition of, 82*t*

if/then statements, 142–143, 142*f*
implicit bias, 73–74
Improving Chronic Illness Care, 20
incidence, definition of term, 8*t*
Information-Motivation-Behavioral skills (IMB), 97
institutional racism
    COVID-19 pandemic and, 171–172
    definition of, 81*t*
    effect on health outcomes, 2
internal consistency, in program evaluation, 145–146
intersectionality
    cultural competency and, 71, 74–75, 169
    definition of, 81*t*

intervention and strategies. *See also* program evaluation
    clinical trials, 123–131, 125*t*
    key points, 135
    patient navigation, 85–100, 88*f*, 89*f*, 91*f*, 93*t*, 94*f*, 95*f*, 99*f*
    survivorship care plans (SCPs), 112–121, 112, 116*b*
intervention research, 158, 159*b*
Islam (Muslim) beliefs and practices, 79
"-Isms," definition of, 82*t*

Jehovah's Witnesses beliefs and practices, 79
Judaism beliefs and practices, 79

language
    considering key stakeholders' preferences, 141
    cultural competency and, 72, 81*t*
    discrimination stress due to, 49
    effect on health literacy, 33, 76
    limited English proficiency (LEP), 32
    linguicism, 82*t*
    plain-language communication, 30, 40*b*, 88
    standards for CLAS, 77
    translation services, 34*b*
LGBTQIA, definition of, 82*t*
limited English proficiency (LEP), 32
linguicism, 82*t*
logic models, 142–143, 142*f*
lung cancer
    causes of and risk factors for, 9
    preventing, 10*t*
    screening recommendations, 11, 12*f*, 12*t*
    types of, 9
Lutheran beliefs and practices, 79

MacColl Center for Health Care Innovation, 20
major lifetime events, 48–49
mammography screening
    CCM components implemented for, 24*t*
    multiple dimensions of influence, 152
    overcoming barriers to, 91–92
    preparation tips, 98*f*
marginalized persons
    addressing challenges faced by, 146
    definition of, 82*t*
    intersectionality and, 74–75
    program assessment, 136, 170
Medicaid expansions, 171
Methodist, United, beliefs and practices, 79
MI (clinical intervention), 5
microaggression, definition of, 82*t*
mortality, definition of term, 8*t*
motivation
    motivational interviewing (MI), 92–95, 93*t*, 94*f*, 95*f*
    OARS (Open-ended questioning, Affirming, Reflecting, and Summarizing) technique, 95–96, 96*f*
Motivation-Behavioral (IMB) skills, 159*b*

National Cancer Institute (NCI)
    effect of social factors on cancer disparities, 4
    funding of clinical trials, 123
    health communication planning process, 36f
    information available from, 66, 92
    number of cancer survivors, 112
    survivorship care plans (SCPs), 115
Native Americans beliefs and practices, 79
Navigation-Information-Motivation-Behavioral
        Skills (NIMBS), 159b
Navigation Information-Motivation-Behavioral
        skills Problem solving (NIMBs-Ps), 97–99, 99f

OARS (Open-ended questioning, Affirming,
        Reflecting, and Summarizing) technique,
        95–96, 96f
obesity
    association with discrimination and bias, 2
    influence on cancer outcomes, 115, 119
oncologists, definition of term, 8t
open-ended questions. See OARS (Open-ended
        questioning, Affirming, Reflecting, and
        Summarizing) technique
oppression
    definition of, 82t
    intersectionality and, 74
outcomes and assessing intervention efforts
    CDC framework for program evaluation, 140f
    cycle of evidence-based public health, 139f
    logic model: if/then statements, 142f
    program evaluation, 136–148

patient navigation
    adapting for high-risk, hard-to-reach
        populations, 97–99, 99f
    beginning the process, 88
    behavioral skills, 97
    concept of, 86
    core principles of, 86–87
    focus areas, 85
    guiding principles, 88f
    information, 91–92
    information sheet, 89f
    motivation, 92–96, 93t, 94f, 95f
    overview of, 169
    problem solving, 89–90, 91f
    stages of, 86
    training for patient navigators, 87–88
patient navigators
    definition of term, 8t
    roles in survivorship care plans, 116b
    training for, 87–88
Patient Protection and Affordable Care Act (ACA),
        31, 86, 168
Pentecostal (Assembly of God, Foursquare Church), 79
policy research, designing and conducting, 158, 159b
poverty profiles
    65-plus years old, 57–58
    chronic poverty, 64–65

female head of household with children, 55–56
homeless women, 61–62
of low-income women, 54–55
racial/ethnic minorities or "underclass," 65–66
rural residents, 60–61
temporary poverty, 63
working poor, 59–60
practice-based research, 137–138
predictive validity, 145–146
prejudice
    definition of, 82t
    exposed through self-assessment, 141
problem funnel, 90, 91f
problem solving, 89–90, 91f
procedural skills, 97
process evaluations, 143
program evaluation
    assessing community strengths and dynamics,
        156–157b
    Body and Soul program, 158f
    CBPR (community-based participatory
        research), 149–163, 151f
    CDC framework for program evaluation, 140f
    community sites participating, 155f
    cycle of evidence-based public health, 139f
    designing and conducting intervention research,
        159b
    focusing research efforts, 153b
    forming partnerships through engagement, 154b
    key points, 166
    logic model: if/then statements, 142f
    maintaining, sustaining, and evaluating CBPR
        partnerships, 160f
    outcomes and assessing intervention efforts,
        136–148
    overview of, 170
    program for elimination of cancer disparities,
        161–162b
Program for the Elimination of Cancer Disparities
        (PECaD), 161–162b
public health evidence, 137–139

qualitative evaluations, 144
quantitative evaluations, 144

race
    changes in race and ethnicity compositions in
        U.S., 76
    culturally competent evaluators and, 141
    definition of, 82t
    effect on cancer/health disparities, 8, 8t, 72, 75–76
    versus ethnicity, 81t
    five-year cancer survival by race and sex, 112t
    health equity and, 2
    self-regulation skills and, 145
    as social determinant of health, 77
racism
    acknowledging, 80
    COVID-19 pandemic and, 2, 171

definition of, 82t
  intersectionality and, 74, 81t
recent life events, 48
reliability, in program evaluation, 145–146
religious beliefs and practices, 78–80
religious bias, 73
research findings
  disseminating and translating, 160
  feeding back and interpreting, 159
risk factors
  for cancer, 9–11, 10t
  cancer navigation and, 38, 54
  cervical cancer screening and, 16, 16f
  for COVID-19, 34b
  CRC (colorectal cancer) screening and, 15
  definition of term, 8t
  evidence-based public health (EBPH) and, 139
  lung cancer screening and, 11
  social determinants of health and, 2–4
Robert Wood Johnson Foundation, 20
Roman Catholic beliefs and practices, 79
Russian Orthodox beliefs and practices, 79

SCP. See survivorship care plans (SCPs)
self-regulation skills, 141, 145–146
SEM (social ecological model), 152
SES. See socioeconomic status (SES)
sexism
  acknowledging, 80
  definition of, 82t
  intersectionality and, 74, 81t
SMART (Specific, Measurable, Achievable,
    Realistic/Relevant, Time Bound) goals,
    141–142
social determinants of health
  cultural competency and, 77
  definition of term, 2, 8t
social disadvantage, definition of term, 8t
social ecological model (SEM), 152
social stressors, influence on cancer outcomes, 115
socioeconomic status (SES)
  CNI scores as indication of, 153b
  culturally competent evaluators and, 141

health equity and, 2
links to cancer and health disparities, 8, 8t,
    75–77
patient navigation and, 86
prejudice based on, 82t
self-regulation skills and, 145
stages of change model, 93
stakeholders
  definition of, 151
  identifying community stakeholders, 151
stereotypes
  avoiding, 141, 144
  definition of, 82t
  implicit bias and, 73, 81t
storyboard illustrations, 127–131
stress exposure list, 48–50
summative evaluations, 143
survivorship care plans (SCPs)
  adapted for socio-ecological areas of relevance,
      117–121
  components of, 113
  continued endorsement of, 114–115
  five-year survival percentage by race and sex, 112
  inconsistent use of, 113
  limited support for, 113–114
  long-term care of cancer survivors, 112
  navigation process and, 87
  overview of, 169
  potential benefits of, 114
  recent criticisms of, 114
  roles for healthcare professionals, 115–116, 116b
  templates for, 113, 115
  usability for minorities, 115
systematic skills, 97

Temporary Assistance for Needy Families (TANF)
      program, 144–145, 170
triple-negative breast cancer subtype, 8

underserved, definition of term, 8t
U.S. Department of Health and Human Services, 19

white privilege, definition of, 82t